The Beauty Secrets

FROM ANCIENT WISDOM TO MODERN SCIENCE - YOUR GUIDE TO TIMELESS BEAUTY

AVELINE SAPHINO

CONTENTS

Introduction

In the bustling corridors of our modern world, the pursuit of beauty is a journey as timeless as the shifting sands of an ancient desert. From the whispered rituals of queens to the promises of glossy advertisements, the quest for beauty has captivated hearts and minds for centuries.

With innovative skincare routines that harness the latest advancements in dermatology, revitalizing hair care regimens, and luxurious body care rituals inspired by ancient traditions, "The Beauty Secrets" is your comprehensive guide to unlocking radiant beauty from head to toe. You'll discover the science behind common skincare concerns such as acne, aging, and hyperpigmentation, and learn how to address them with targeted treatments and routines.

Drawing upon ancient traditions from diverse cultures and blending them with modern insights, this book offers ayurvedic rituals, herbal remedies, mindfulness practices.

You will embark on a journey of self-exploration, uncovering the sacred rituals and practices that have nourished body, mind, and soul for generations.

Let's begin to unlock the radiant beauty that has always been yours to claim!

No more hard work than look beautiful with eight in the morning until midnight.

Brigitte Bardot

LOVE YOURSELF FIRST

Importance Of Skincare And Self-Care

In a world that often moves at a rapid pace, the significance of skincare and self-care cannot be overstated. Beyond the pursuit of outward beauty, these practices are integral to our overall well-being, both physically and emotionally. Skincare serves as a foundation for self-care, offering a tangible way to nurture the body and mind. The history of skincare can be traced back to ancient civilizations, where various cultures developed their own beauty rituals and skincare practices. The evolution of skincare has been influenced by cultural, social, and scientific developments.

Ancient Egyptians were known for their elaborate beauty rituals. They used natural ingredients such as oils, honey, and plant extracts for skincare. Cleopatra, the famous Egyptian queen, was believed to have employed milk baths for her skin. Both ancient Greeks and Romans practiced skincare using a combination of natural ingredients, including olive oil and honey. They also used a variety of masks and scrubs to maintain healthy skin.

During the Middle Ages, skincare practices were influenced by religious beliefs, and cosmetics were often associated with vanity. The Renaissance period saw a revival of interest in beauty, with women using various concoctions and powders to achieve a pale complexion.

The 19th century was the start of mass-produced cosmetics. Cold creams and rouges became popular during this time. The beauty industry began to commercialize skincare products, making them more accessible to a broader audience. The emergence of well-known skincare brands and the development of more advanced formulations happened later. Cold creams, cleansers, and moisturizers became standard parts of skincare routines. In the mid-20th century, advancements in dermatology and skincare science led to the development of ingredients like retinoids and alpha hydroxy acids (AHAs). These ingredients revolutionized anti-aging skincare.

The latter half of the century also saw increased awareness of sun protection, with the introduction of sunscreens to prevent skin damage from UV rays.

The 21st century has seen a surge in skincare innovations and technology. Ingredients like hyaluronic acid, peptides, and antioxidants are commonly used in skincare products.

The rise of social media has contributed to the popularity of skincare, with information and product recommendations readily shared online. This has led to a more educated consumer base and a growing global skincare market.

Personalized skincare routines, incorporating products tailored to individual skin concerns, have become increasingly popular. Advances in genetic testing and skincare technology also contribute to this trend.

Skincare rituals can extend beyond the practical aspects of cleansing and moisturizing. They become personal moments of self-care, providing a pause in the hustle and bustle of our routines. These rituals, whether it's a soothing face mask at the end of a long day or a rejuvenating morning routine, offer a chance to reconnect with oneself, fostering a positive relationship with our bodies. Focusing on the present moment while applying skincare products allows us to cultivate a sense of awareness and relaxation, acknowledge our own value and prioritize health and happiness.

Consistent skincare practices contribute to the prevention of common skin concerns such as acne, pigmentation, and premature aging. By prioritizing skincare, we can lay the foundation for long-term skin health, minimizing the need for corrective measures later in life.

UNDERSTANDING YOUR SKIN. THE BASICS OF A SKINCARE ROUTINE BY SKIN TYPES

Different Skin Types And Concerns

The classification of skin types is typically based on factors such as oil production, sensitivity, and susceptibility to various skin conditions. The most common skin types are:

Normal skin:
Characteristics: Well-balanced, neither too oily nor too dry.

Traits: Fine pores, smooth texture, good blood circulation, and a healthy complexion.

Dry skin:
Characteristics: Lacks sufficient oil (sebum) production, leading to a tight or flaky feel.

Traits: Small pores, dull complexion, may be prone to fine lines and wrinkles.

Oily skin:
Characteristics: Overactive sebaceous glands produce excess oil.

Traits: Large pores, shiny or greasy complexion, prone to acne and blackheads.

Combination skin:
Characteristics: Combination of different skin types on different areas of the face.

Traits: T-zone (forehead, nose, and chin) may be oily, while cheeks and eye areas can be normal or dry.

Sensitive skin:
Characteristics: Prone to irritation, redness, or reactions to certain products or environmental factors.

Traits: May react adversely to harsh skincare ingredients, fragrances, or extreme weather conditions.

Acne-prone skin:
Characteristics: Pores are more likely to become clogged, leading to the development of acne and blemishes.
Traits: Often associated with excess oil production and inflammation.

Mature or aging skin:
Characteristics: Loss of elasticity, fine lines, wrinkles, and decreased collagen production.
Traits: Requires extra hydration and may benefit from anti-aging ingredients like retinol and antioxidants.

Normal to sensitive skin:
Characteristics: Combination of normal and sensitive traits.
Traits: Skin may be generally well-balanced but is prone to irritation or reactions to certain products.
It's important to note that individuals may experience changes in their skin type due to factors such as age, weather, hormones, and skincare habits.

Additionally, skin concerns like dehydration, sun damage, and environmental exposure can affect overall skin health. Adjusting your skincare routine based on your skin's current needs can help maintain a healthy complexion. If you have specific skin concerns or conditions, consulting with a dermatologist can provide personalized guidance.

Normal skin type

Normal skin is considered the ideal skin type, characterized by a well-balanced state of oil production, moisture retention, and a generally healthy complexion. People with normal skin often experience minimal skin concerns, and their skin tends to be versatile and adaptable to various skincare products. Here's a detailed look at normal skin:

Balanced oil production: Normal skin has a healthy balance of oil (sebum) production. The sebaceous glands produce just enough oil to keep the skin moisturized without making it excessively oily.

Even texture and tone: The texture of normal skin is generally smooth and even. Pores are not enlarged, and there is no excessive dryness or oiliness. Normal skin often has a natural, radiant glow.

Good blood circulation: Normal skin is characterized by good blood circulation, contributing to a healthy and vibrant appearance. This skin type typically has adequate oxygen and nutrient supply.

Few skin concerns: Individuals with normal skin types typically experience minimal skin concerns. They may not face issues such as excessive dryness, oiliness, or sensitivity.

Skincare routine for normal skin:

While normal skin requires less intensive care than other skin types, maintaining a consistent skincare routine is important for preserving its balanced state and preventing potential issues. A basic skincare routine for normal skin may include:

Cleansing: Use a gentle, hydrating cleanser to remove impurities without stripping the skin of its natural oils. Cleansing can be done morning and night.

Toning: Apply a mild, alcohol-free toner to balance the skin's pH levels and prepare it for subsequent products.

Moisturizing: Even though normal skin doesn't usually suffer from dryness, a lightweight moisturizer can help maintain hydration and support the skin's barrier function.

Sunscreen: Protect normal skin from sun damage by using a broad-spectrum sunscreen with at least SPF 30. Sunscreen should be applied daily, even on cloudy days.

Treatment (if needed): Depending on individual concerns, normal skin may benefit from occasional treatments such as exfoliation or masks. However, these are not necessary for daily use.

Tips for normal skin:

Experiment with products: People with normal skin have the flexibility to experiment with different skincare products. However, it's still important to patch-test new products to ensure compatibility.

Adjust to seasons: Normal skin may experience slight changes with the seasons. Adjust your skincare routine accordingly, such as using a slightly richer moisturizer in colder months.

Stay hydrated and maintain a healthy lifestyle: Drinking enough water and adopting a healthy lifestyle with balanced nutrition can contribute to maintaining normal skin health.

While normal skin may not require intensive care, it's crucial to tailor your skincare routine to individual preferences and any specific concerns that may arise over time. Regular maintenance and protection are key to preserving the natural balance and vibrancy of normal skin.

Dry skin type

Dry skin is characterized by a lack of moisture and oil (sebum) on the skin's surface. This skin type can be influenced by various factors, including genetics, environmental conditions, and age. Dry skin is prone to feeling tight, rough, and may exhibit signs of flakiness or scaling. Here's a detailed look at dry skin:

Lack of sebum production: Dry skin is often the result of underactive sebaceous glands that produce insufficient sebum. Sebum helps to retain moisture and protect the skin.

Tightness and roughness: Dry skin can feel tight, especially after cleansing, and may have a rough or uneven texture. The lack of adequate moisture can lead to discomfort.

Flakiness and scaling: Dry skin is prone to flakiness and scaling, especially in areas such as the cheeks and forehead. This can become more noticeable when the skin is dry or exposed to harsh environmental conditions.

Dull appearance: Dry skin may appear dull or lack the natural radiance seen in well-hydrated skin. The lack of moisture can contribute to a less vibrant complexion.

Fine lines and wrinkles: Dry skin is more prone to the early development of fine lines and wrinkles. The reduced moisture levels can accentuate the appearance of aging.

Causes of dry skin:

Genetics: Some individuals may be genetically predisposed to dry skin, inheriting a tendency for underactive sebaceous glands.

Environmental factors: Exposure to dry or cold climates, low humidity, or harsh winds can contribute to skin dryness.

Age: Aging is associated with a decrease in sebum production, making the skin more prone to dryness and wrinkles.

Hot water and harsh cleansers: Excessive use of hot water and harsh cleansers can strip the skin of its natural oils, exacerbating dryness.

Certain medical conditions: Conditions such as eczema, psoriasis, or hypothyroidism can contribute to dry skin.

Skincare routine for dry skin:

An effective skincare routine for dry skin focuses on hydration and barrier repair. Here's a recommended routine:

Gentle cleansing: Use a mild, hydrating cleanser to cleanse the skin without stripping away natural oils. Avoid hot water and opt for lukewarm temperatures.

Hydrating toner: Apply a hydrating toner to replenish moisture and prepare the skin for subsequent products.

Hydrating serum: Incorporate a hyaluronic acid serum to boost hydration. This ingredient attracts and retains water, helping to plump and moisturize the skin.

Rich moisturizer: Choose a rich, emollient moisturizer to lock in moisture. Look for ingredients like shea butter, ceramides, and fatty acids.

Sunscreen: Protect dry skin from sun damage with a broad-spectrum sunscreen with at least SPF 30. Opt for a moisturizing sunscreen formula.

Occasional exfoliation: Exfoliate the skin 1-2 times a week with a gentle exfoliant to remove dead skin cells and promote cell turnover. Avoid harsh scrubs.

Hydrating masks: Use hydrating masks or overnight masks to provide an extra boost of moisture as needed.

Tips for dry skin:

Stay hydrated: Drink plenty of water to hydrate the skin from within.

Humidifier: Use a humidifier in dry indoor environments to add moisture to the air.

Avoid harsh products: Steer clear of products with alcohol, fragrances, and harsh chemicals, as they can exacerbate dryness.

Diet: Consume foods rich in omega-3 fatty acids and antioxidants to support skin health.

Consult a dermatologist: If dryness persists or worsens, consult a dermatologist for personalized advice and potential treatment options.

Tailoring your skincare routine to address the specific needs of dry skin is essential for restoring moisture, improving comfort, and maintaining a healthy complexion.

Oily skin type

Oily skin is characterized by an overproduction of sebum, the skin's natural oil. This excess oil can lead to a shiny complexion, enlarged pores, and an increased susceptibility to acne and blackheads. While oily skin has its challenges, it also has certain benefits, such as delayed signs of aging. Here's a detailed look at oily skin:

Excess sebum production: Oily skin is characterized by an overactive sebaceous gland, resulting in an excess production of sebum. This can create a shiny appearance, particularly in the T-zone (forehead, nose, and chin).

Enlarged pores: Oily skin is often associated with larger pores. The excess oil production can contribute to the dilation of pores, making them more visible.

Shiny complexion: Due to the surplus of oil on the skin's surface, individuals with oily skin may experience a persistent shine, especially in the central part of the face.

Acne and blackheads: Oily skin is more prone to acne breakouts and the formation of blackheads (open comedones) due to the increased likelihood of pores becoming clogged with excess oil and dead skin cells.

Delayed signs of aging: Oily skin tends to show fewer early signs of aging, such as fine lines and wrinkles, compared to drier skin types. The natural oils can act as a protective barrier.

Causes of oily skin:

Genetics: Genetic factors play a role in determining skin type, and individuals with a family history of oily skin may be more prone to it.

Hormones: Hormonal fluctuations, especially during puberty, menstruation, and pregnancy, can contribute to increased sebum production.

Climate: Hot and humid climates can stimulate sebum production. Oily skin may be more prominent in regions with such weather conditions.

Overuse of harsh products: Paradoxically, using harsh cleansers or products that strip the skin of oil can trigger an overcompensation in sebum production.

Skincare routine for oily skin:

A balanced skincare routine for oily skin focuses on controlling excess oil while maintaining hydration. Here's a recommended routine:

Gentle cleansing: Use a gentle, foaming cleanser to remove excess oil and impurities without over-drying the skin. Cleansing twice a day is typically recommended.

Oil-free toner: Apply an alcohol-free, oil-free toner to help balance the skin's pH and remove any remaining traces of oil or debris.

Lightweight moisturizer: Even oily skin needs hydration. Choose a lightweight, non-comedogenic moisturizer to provide hydration without clogging pores.

Oil-free sunscreen: Protect the skin from UV damage with an oil-free, broad-spectrum sunscreen with at least SPF 30. Look for formulations designed for oily or acne-prone skin.

Salicylic acid or glycolic acid: Incorporate a chemical exfoliant containing salicylic acid or glycolic acid 2-3 times a week to help unclog pores and promote cell turnover.

Clay masks: Use clay masks once a week to absorb excess oil and reduce shine. Kaolin or bentonite clay can be beneficial.

Avoid heavy makeup: Opt for oil-free, non-comedogenic makeup products to avoid further clogging of pores.

Tips for oily skin:

Consistent cleansing: Regular cleansing helps control excess oil. However, avoid overwashing, as this can trigger more oil production.

Blotting papers: Keep blotting papers or oil-absorbing sheets on hand to manage excess oil throughout the day.

Hydration: Don't skip moisturizer, as even oily skin needs hydration. Choose oil-free, water-based formulations.

Limit touching: Avoid touching the face excessively, as this can transfer oils and contribute to breakouts.

Consult a dermatologist: If oily skin is accompanied by persistent acne or other skin concerns, consult a dermatologist for personalized advice and potential treatments.

Balancing the oil production of oily skin involves finding the right combination of products and habits. Consistency in skincare practices is key to maintaining healthy and balanced oily skin.

Combination skin type

Combination skin is characterized by having a mix of different skin types on different areas of the face. Typically, individuals with combination skin experience both oily and dry or normal areas. The most common combination is an oily T-zone (forehead, nose, and chin) with drier or normal cheeks. Managing combination skin involves addressing the unique needs of each area. Here's a detailed look at combination skin:

Oily t-zone: The forehead, nose, and chin (T-zone) tend to be oilier due to higher sebum production and larger pores.

Normal or dry cheeks: The cheeks and eye areas may experience normal to dry skin, with potential signs of tightness or flakiness.

Enlarged pores: The pores in the T-zone may appear larger due to increased oil production, while the pores on the cheeks may be smaller.

Occasional breakouts: Individuals with combination skin may experience occasional breakouts, particularly in the oily areas.

Seasonal changes: Combination skin can exhibit variations in different seasons, with the T-zone becoming more oily in hot and humid conditions, and the cheek areas feeling drier in colder weather.

Causes of combination skin:

Genetics: Genetic factors can contribute to combination skin, with certain families having a predisposition to varied skin types.

Hormones: Hormonal fluctuations, especially during puberty, menstruation, and pregnancy, can affect sebum production and contribute to combination skin.

Climate: Environmental factors, such as changes in weather and humidity levels, can impact the skin differently in various areas.

Skincare habits: Overusing products targeted for one specific skin type or using harsh cleansers can disrupt the skin's balance, leading to combination skin.

Skincare routine for combination skin:

Managing combination skin involves finding a balance between addressing oiliness in the T-zone and providing adequate hydration to drier areas. Here's a recommended routine:

Gentle cleansing: Use a mild, hydrating cleanser to remove impurities without over-drying the skin. Cleansing twice a day is typically recommended.

Balancing toner: Apply a toner to balance the skin's ph levels and address excess oil in the T-zone while providing hydration to drier areas.

Hydrating serum: Incorporate a hydrating serum with ingredients like hyaluronic acid to provide moisture to drier areas without making oily areas greasier.

Lightweight moisturizer: Use a lightweight, non-comedogenic moisturizer that caters to both dry and oily areas. Apply more moisturizer on drier areas and less on oilier regions.

Sunscreen: Protect the skin from UV damage with a broad-spectrum sunscreen with at least SPF 30. Choose a sunscreen suitable for combination skin.

Exfoliation: Use a chemical exfoliant containing salicylic acid or glycolic acid 1-2 times a week to address clogged pores and promote cell turnover.

Spot treatment (if needed): For occasional breakouts, use targeted spot treatments on specific areas rather than applying all over the face.

Tips for combination skin:

Customize products: Tailor your skincare routine based on the specific needs of different areas. Use products designed for combination skin.

Seasonal adjustments: Adjust your skincare routine according to seasonal changes. In colder months, you may need to add more hydration, while in warmer months, focus on controlling excess oil.

Avoid harsh ingredients: Steer clear of harsh cleansers or products that may strip the skin of its natural oils, as this can exacerbate combination skin.

Consult a dermatologist: If you find it challenging to manage combination skin or if you have specific concerns, consult a dermatologist for personalized advice and product recommendations.

Finding the right balance in your skincare routine is crucial for managing combination skin effectively. Paying attention to the specific needs of each area and adapting your routine accordingly will help maintain a harmonious and healthy complexion.

Sensitive skin type

Sensitive skin is characterized by a heightened reactivity to external factors, resulting in redness, irritation, and discomfort. Individuals with sensitive skin may experience reactions to various skincare products, environmental factors, or specific ingredients. Managing sensitive skin involves using gentle, hypoallergenic products and adopting a careful approach to skincare. Here's a detailed look at sensitive skin:

Redness and irritation: Sensitive skin is prone to redness and irritation, often triggered by environmental factors, certain ingredients, or harsh products.

Tightness and discomfort: Individuals with sensitive skin may experience sensations of tightness, itching, burning, or stinging, especially after using certain skincare products.

Reactivity to products: Sensitive skin reacts adversely to many skincare and cosmetic products, leading to allergic reactions, contact dermatitis, or other forms of irritation.

Vulnerable to environmental factors: Sensitive skin is more vulnerable to environmental factors such as sun exposure, wind, and extreme temperatures, which can exacerbate redness and irritation.

Prone to allergies: People with sensitive skin may have allergies to certain ingredients commonly found in skincare products, fragrances, preservatives, or dyes.

Causes of sensitive skin:

Genetics: Genetic predisposition can play a role in the development of sensitive skin. If your family has a history of sensitive skin, you may be more prone to it.

Skin conditions: Certain skin conditions, such as eczema, rosacea, or contact dermatitis, can contribute to increased skin sensitivity.

Allergies: Allergies to specific ingredients or environmental factors can cause skin sensitivity.

Harsh products: The use of harsh skincare products, including those with strong fragrances or alcohol, can strip the skin's natural protective barrier, leading to sensitivity.

Environmental factors: Exposure to harsh weather conditions, pollution, or UV rays can exacerbate sensitivity.

Skincare routine for sensitive skin:

When creating a skincare routine for sensitive skin, it's important to use gentle, fragrance-free products that won't irritate or exacerbate sensitivity. Here's a basic skincare routine tailored for sensitive skin:

Cleanser: Use a gentle, fragrance-free cleanser formulated for sensitive skin. Look for non-foaming or cream cleansers that are free of harsh ingredients such as sulfates and alcohol. Avoid hot water, as it can further strip the skin of its natural oils. Cleanse your face morning and evening to remove dirt, oil, and impurities without causing irritation.

Toner (optional): If you choose to use a toner, opt for an alcohol-free soothing toner designed for sensitive skin. Look for ingredients like witch hazel, rose water, or chamomile extract that help hydrate and calm the skin. Apply the toner to a cotton pad and gently swipe it over your face after cleansing.

Moisturizer: Select a gentle, fragrance-free moisturizer specifically formulated for sensitive skin. Look for lightweight, non-comedogenic formulas that provide hydration without clogging pores or causing irritation. Ingredients like hyaluronic acid, ceramides, and glycerin can help soothe and replenish the skin's moisture barrier. Apply the moisturizer to damp skin morning and evening to lock in hydration.

Sunscreen: Protect your sensitive skin from harmful UV rays by applying a broad-spectrum sunscreen with SPF 30 or higher every morning, regardless of the weather. Choose a mineral sunscreen containing zinc oxide or titanium dioxide, which are less likely to cause irritation than chemical sunscreens. Apply sunscreen generously to all exposed areas of skin and reapply every two hours when outdoors.

Night cream (optional): If desired, use a gentle, nourishing night cream to help repair and replenish your skin while you sleep. Look for formulations containing soothing ingredients like niacinamide, shea butter, or oat extract to calm and hydrate sensitive skin. Apply the night cream to clean, dry skin before bedtime.

Weekly treatments (optional): Incorporate gentle, non-abrasive exfoliation and masking treatments into your skincare routine on a weekly basis. Choose products specifically formulated for sensitive skin and avoid harsh physical exfoliants or chemical peels that can cause irritation. Opt for mild exfoliants like enzyme masks or gentle scrubs with round beads to slough away dead skin cells without aggravating sensitivity.

Patch test new products: Before introducing new skincare products into your routine, perform a patch test on a small area of skin to check for any adverse reactions or irritation. Apply a small amount of the product to the inside of your wrist or behind your ear and wait 24-48 hours to see if any redness, itching, or inflammation occurs.

Remember to listen to your skin and adjust your skincare routine as needed based on its individual needs and sensitivities. If you experience persistent or severe irritation, consult with a dermatologist for personalized recommendations and treatment options.

Opt for products with minimal ingredients to reduce the likelihood of allergic reactions. Look for formulas with soothing ingredients like calendula, chamomile, or aloe vera. Protect sensitive skin from UV damage with a hypoallergenic, broad-spectrum sunscreen with at least SPF 30. Limit exfoliation to once a week with a mild, non-abrasive exfoliant to avoid exacerbating sensitivity.

Tips for sensitive skin:

Avoid hot water: Use lukewarm water for cleansing and bathing, as hot water can strip the skin of its natural oils.

Protect from environmental factors: Shield sensitive skin from harsh weather conditions by wearing appropriate clothing and using protective measures like hats and sunscreen.

Consult a dermatologist: If you have persistent sensitivity or skin conditions, consult a dermatologist for personalized advice and potential treatment options.

Keep it simple: Adopt a minimalist approach to skincare, focusing on gentle, nourishing products with few ingredients.

Stay hydrated: Adequate hydration is crucial for sensitive skin. Drink plenty of water to maintain skin health from within.

Caring for sensitive skin involves a careful selection of products and a gentle approach to skincare. Avoiding potential triggers and using soothing, hypoallergenic formulations can help manage sensitivity and maintain a calm and healthy complexion.

Acne-prone skin

Acne-prone skin is characterized by a tendency to develop various types of acne lesions, including blackheads, whiteheads, pimples, and cysts. This skin type is often associated with increased sebum production, clogged pores, and inflammation. Managing acne-prone skin involves a targeted skincare routine, lifestyle adjustments, and, in some cases, professional intervention. Here's a detailed look at acne-prone skin:

Excess sebum production: Acne-prone skin tends to produce an excess of sebum (oil). This overproduction can lead to clogged pores and the development of acne lesions.

Clogged pores: Pores in acne-prone skin are more likely to become clogged with a combination of sebum, dead skin cells, and bacteria, leading to the formation of blackheads and whiteheads.

Inflammation: Inflammatory acne, characterized by red and swollen lesions, is common in acne-prone skin. Pimples, papules, and cysts may result from the inflammatory response.

Types of acne lesions:

Blackheads (open comedones): Open pores filled with oxidized sebum and dead skin cells.

Whiteheads (closed comedones): Closed pores containing trapped sebum and debris beneath the skin's surface.

Papules: Small, red, inflamed bumps.

Pustules: Red bumps with a white or yellow center filled with pus.

Nodules: Large, painful lumps beneath the skin's surface.

Cysts: Deep, inflamed, pus-filled lesions that can be painful and leave scars.

Causes of acne-prone skin:

Hormones: Hormonal fluctuations, especially during puberty, menstruation, and pregnancy, play a significant role in acne development.

Genetics: A family history of acne can increase the likelihood of developing acne-prone skin.

Excess sebum production: Overactive sebaceous glands produce more sebum, contributing to clogged pores and acne lesions.

Bacteria: The presence of Propionibacterium acnes (P. acnes) bacteria on the skin can contribute to inflammation and acne.

Dietary factors: Certain dietary factors, such as a high glycemic index diet and dairy consumption, may influence acne.

Stress: Stress can exacerbate acne by triggering hormonal changes and increasing sebum production.

Skincare routine for acne-prone skin:

An effective skincare routine for acne-prone skin aims to manage excess oil, prevent clogged pores, and reduce inflammation. Here's a recommended routine:

Gentle cleansing: Use a mild, non-comedogenic cleanser to cleanse the skin twice a day, especially after sweating.

Salicylic acid cleanser: Incorporate a salicylic acid cleanser 2-3 times a week to exfoliate and help unclog pores.

Oil-free and non-comedogenic products: Choose oil-free and non-comedogenic moisturizers, sunscreens, and makeup to avoid clogging pores.

Non-comedogenic makeup: Use makeup labeled as non-comedogenic to prevent pore blockage.

Benzoyl peroxide or salicylic acid treatment: Apply a spot treatment containing benzoyl peroxide or salicylic acid directly on acne lesions to help reduce inflammation.

Oil-free sunscreen: Protect the skin from UV damage with a broad-spectrum, oil-free sunscreen with at least SPF 30.

Avoid harsh scrubs: Avoid abrasive scrubs, as they can irritate the skin and worsen acne lesions.

Tips for acne-prone skin:

Hands off: Avoid picking or squeezing acne lesions, as this can lead to scarring and worsen inflammation.

Hydration: Stay hydrated to maintain overall skin health, but choose water-based moisturizers to avoid excess oil.

Regular cleaning: Wash pillowcases, hats, and other items that come in contact with the face regularly to prevent bacterial buildup.

Limit dairy and high glycemic foods: Consider reducing the intake of dairy and high glycemic index foods.

Mature or aging skin

Mature or aging skin refers to skin that has undergone natural aging processes, resulting in changes such as loss of elasticity, wrinkles, fine lines, and a decrease in collagen and elastin production. While aging is a natural and inevitable part of life, skincare practices can help minimize the visible signs of aging and maintain healthy, radiant skin. Here's a detailed look at mature or aging skin:

Loss of elasticity: Aging skin experiences a decline in the production of collagen and elastin, leading to a loss of skin elasticity and firmness.

Wrinkles and fine lines: The appearance of wrinkles and fine lines is a common characteristic of aging skin. These lines may develop around the eyes, mouth, and forehead.

Thinning of the skin: Aging skin often becomes thinner, making blood vessels more visible and increasing susceptibility to bruising.

Uneven skin tone: Hyperpigmentation (dark spots) and uneven skin tone may become more noticeable as aging skin may have accumulated sun damage over the years.

Dryness: Mature skin tends to be drier as oil production decreases, leading to increased susceptibility to dryness and dehydration.

Decreased collagen production: Collagen, a protein responsible for skin structure, decreases with age, contributing to the formation of wrinkles and sagging.

Decreased cell turnover: The rate of skin cell turnover decreases, leading to a slower renewal process and a duller complexion.

Causes of aging skin:

Intrinsic aging: This refers to the natural aging process influenced by genetics, which determines factors like skin thickness and collagen production.

Extrinsic aging: Environmental factors play a significant role in aging skin. Sun exposure, pollution, smoking, and other lifestyle choices contribute to premature aging.

Hormonal changes: Changes in hormone levels, particularly during menopause, can impact the skin's structure and moisture retention.

Lack of skincare: Neglecting skincare routines, including inadequate sun protection, can accelerate the aging process.

Skincare routine for mature or aging skin:

A skincare routine for mature or aging skin focuses on hydration, collagen stimulation, and protection against further damage. Here's a recommended routine:

Gentle cleansing: Use a mild, hydrating cleanser to clean the skin without stripping away essential moisture. Avoid harsh soaps.

Hydrating toner: Apply a hydrating toner with ingredients like hyaluronic acid to replenish moisture and prepare the skin for subsequent products.

Antioxidant serum: Incorporate an antioxidant-rich serum containing ingredients like vitamin C to protect the skin from free radical damage.

Collagen-boosting ingredients: Use products with ingredients known to stimulate collagen production, such as retinoids (retinol) and peptides.

Moisturizing cream: Choose a rich, nourishing moisturizer to address dryness and support the skin's barrier function. Look for ingredients like ceramides and fatty acids.

Sunscreen: Protect mature skin from further sun damage with a broad-spectrum sunscreen with at least SPF 30. Sunscreen is crucial for preventing premature aging.

Exfoliation: Include gentle exfoliation 1-2 times a week to promote cell turnover. Use chemical exfoliants like alpha hydroxy acids (AHAs) or beta hydroxy acids (BHAs).

Eye cream: Use a specialized eye cream to address concerns such as crow's feet and under-eye wrinkles.

Tips for mature or aging skin:

Stay hydrated: Drink plenty of water to maintain skin hydration from within.

Healthy lifestyle: Adopt a healthy lifestyle with a balanced diet, regular exercise, and adequate sleep to support overall well-being, which reflects in the skin.

Avoid smoking: Smoking accelerates aging, leading to wrinkles and a dull complexion. Quitting smoking can have positive effects on the skin.

Consult a dermatologist: If you have specific concerns or are considering more advanced treatments, consult a dermatologist for personalized advice and potential treatments like laser therapy or injectables.

Taking a proactive and consistent approach to skincare is essential for maintaining the health and appearance of mature or aging skin. A combination of protective measures, hydration, and targeted treatments can contribute to a more youthful and radiant complexion.

Normal to sensitive skin

Normal to sensitive skin is a combination skin type that exhibits characteristics of both normal and sensitive skin. While the skin is generally well-balanced, individuals with normal to sensitive skin may experience occasional sensitivity, redness, or reactions to certain products. Managing this skin type involves using gentle products that maintain the overall health of the skin without causing irritation. Here's a detailed look at normal to sensitive skin:

Well-Balanced: The skin is generally well-balanced, with normal oil production and a smooth, even texture.

Occasional sensitivity: Individuals with normal to sensitive skin may experience occasional sensitivity, redness, or irritation, especially in response to certain skincare products or environmental factors.

Vulnerable to irritants: The skin may be more susceptible to reactions from harsh ingredients, fragrances, or environmental aggressors, leading to temporary sensitivity.

Normal texture and pores: The skin has a normal texture with neither excessive dryness nor oiliness. Pores are typically not enlarged.

Responsive to weather changes: Normal to sensitive skin may show variations in sensitivity based on changes in weather or environmental conditions.

Causes of normal to sensitive skin:

Genetics: Genetic factors can contribute to the skin's sensitivity, with some individuals having a natural predisposition to occasional redness or irritation.

Environmental factors: Exposure to harsh weather conditions, pollution, or UV rays can trigger sensitivity in individuals with normal to sensitive skin.

Product sensitivity: The use of skincare products containing harsh ingredients, fragrances, or allergens may lead to temporary sensitivity.

Climate changes: Changes in climate, such as transitioning from a humid to a dry environment, can affect the skin's balance.

Skincare routine for normal to sensitive skin:

Managing normal to sensitive skin involves using gentle, soothing products that maintain balance without causing irritation. Here's a recommended routine:

Gentle cleansing: Use a mild, fragrance-free cleanser to clean the skin without stripping away natural oils. Cleansing twice a day is typically recommended.

Alcohol-free toner: Apply an alcohol-free, soothing toner with calming ingredients like chamomile or aloe vera to help balance the skin's pH and provide hydration.

Hypoallergenic moisturizer: Choose a hypoallergenic, fragrance-free moisturizer that provides hydration without clogging pores or causing irritation.

Fragrance-free products: Opt for skincare products labeled as fragrance-free to minimize the risk of irritation.

Sunscreen: Protect the skin from UV damage with a broad-spectrum sunscreen with at least SPF 30. Choose a sunscreen suitable for sensitive skin.

Avoid harsh exfoliation: Limit exfoliation to once a week with a mild, non-abrasive exfoliant to avoid exacerbating sensitivity.

Patch test new products: Before introducing new products into your routine, conduct patch tests to check for any adverse reactions.

Tips for normal to sensitive skin:

Allergy testing: If you suspect specific ingredients trigger sensitivity, consider allergy testing to identify potential allergens.

Environmental protection: Shield the skin from harsh weather conditions by wearing protective clothing and using sunscreen.

Stay hydrated: Drink enough water to maintain skin hydration from within.

Cool compresses: If temporary sensitivity occurs, applying cool compresses can help soothe the skin.

Consult a dermatologist: If sensitivity persists or worsens, consult a dermatologist for personalized advice and potential treatments.

Balancing normal to sensitive skin involves using a gentle skincare routine that caters to the skin's occasional sensitivity without compromising its overall health. Paying attention to environmental factors and using hypoallergenic products can help maintain a calm and well-nourished complexion.

Common Skin Concerns And How To Address Them

1. Acne

Cause: Excess sebum production, clogged pores, bacteria, and hormonal fluctuations can contribute to acne.

For acne-prone skin, it's important to establish a comprehensive skincare routine that includes treatments aimed at controlling breakouts, reducing inflammation, and preventing future acne flare-ups.

Here are some effective treatments for acne-prone skin:

Salicylic acid cleanser:
Use a cleanser containing salicylic acid, a beta hydroxy acid (BHA) that helps unclog pores, remove excess oil, and exfoliate dead skin cells. Use it twice daily to keep pores clear and prevent breakouts.

Benzoyl peroxide spot treatment:
Benzoyl peroxide is a potent acne-fighting ingredient that kills acne-causing bacteria, reduces inflammation, and helps unclog pores. Apply benzoyl peroxide spot treatment to active breakouts once or twice daily.

Glycolic Acid or Lactic Acid Exfoliant:
Incorporate a chemical exfoliant containing glycolic acid or lactic acid into your skincare routine. These alpha hydroxy acids (AHAs) help remove dead skin cells, unclog pores, and improve overall skin texture. Use it 2-3 times per week to prevent breakouts and promote cell turnover.

Topical retinoids:
Topical retinoids, such as adapalene, tretinoin, or tazarotene, are prescription-strength treatments that help unclog pores, reduce inflammation, and prevent acne formation. Apply a pea-sized amount of

opical retinoid to clean, dry skin before bedtime, and use it as directed by your dermatologist.

Antibacterial face masks:

Use antibacterial face masks containing ingredients like sulfur, clay, or charcoal once or twice a week to help absorb excess oil, reduce inflammation, and kill acne-causing bacteria. Leave the mask on for 10-15 minutes before rinsing off with lukewarm water.

Oil-free moisturizer:

Use an oil-free, non-comedogenic moisturizer to hydrate your skin without clogging pores. Look for lightweight formulas labeled "oil-free" or "non-comedogenic" to avoid exacerbating acne.

Sunscreen:

Apply a broad-spectrum sunscreen with SPF 30 or higher every morning to protect your skin from harmful UV rays. Look for oil-free or non-comedogenic sunscreens specifically formulated for acne-prone skin.

Professional treatments:

Consider professional acne treatments performed by a dermatologist, such as chemical peels, microdermabrasion, or laser therapy. These treatments can help improve acne symptoms and minimize scarring.

Healthy lifestyle habits:

Maintain a healthy lifestyle by eating a balanced diet, staying hydrated, getting enough sleep, and managing stress levels. These lifestyle factors can influence your skin health and contribute to acne flare-ups.

Remember to be patient and consistent with your skincare routine, as it may take several weeks to see significant improvements in acne-prone skin. If over-the-counter treatments are not effective, consult with a dermatologist for personalized recommendations and prescription-strength medications.

2. Hyperpigmentation

Cause: Hyperpigmentation occurs when there is an overproduction of melanin in certain areas of the skin, leading to dark spots or patches. There are several treatments available to help reduce the appearance of hyperpigmentation and even out skin tone.

Here are some effective treatments for hyperpigmentation:

Topical Lightening Agents:

Topical treatments containing ingredients such as hydroquinone, kojic acid, arbutin, licorice extract, vitamin C, niacinamide (vitamin B3), and alpha hydroxy acids (AHAs) can help lighten dark spots and even out skin tone. These ingredients work by inhibiting melanin production or promoting cell turnover to reveal brighter, more uniform skin.

Retinoids:

Prescription-strength retinoids, such as tretinoin (Retin-A) or adapalene (Differin), can help improve hyperpigmentation by promoting cell turnover, increasing collagen production, and fading dark spots over time. Start with a lower concentration and gradually increase as tolerated to minimize irritation.

Chemical peels:

Chemical peels, such as glycolic acid peels, lactic acid peels, or trichloroacetic acid (TCA) peels, help exfoliate the outer layer of the skin, promoting cell turnover and reducing the appearance of hyperpigmentation. Professional chemical peels performed by a dermatologist or licensed esthetician can provide more dramatic results than at-home peels.

Microdermabrasion:

Microdermabrasion is a non-invasive exfoliating treatment that uses a diamond-tipped wand or crystals to gently remove the outer layer of the skin, helping to fade dark spots and improve skin texture. Multiple sessions may be needed to achieve desired results.

Laser therapy:

Laser therapy, such as intense pulsed light (IPL) or fractional laser resurfacing, can target melanin pigments in the skin and break them down, leading to a reduction in hyperpigmentation. Laser treatments are typically performed by a dermatologist and may require multiple sessions for optimal results.

Microneedling:

Microneedling, also known as collagen induction therapy, involves using tiny needles to create micro-injuries in the skin, stimulating collagen production and improving the appearance of hyperpigmentation. Microneedling can be combined with topical lightening agents or platelet-rich plasma (PRP) for enhanced results.

Sunscreen:
Sun protection is essential for preventing further hyperpigmentation and protecting the skin from UV damage. Apply a broad-spectrum sunscreen with SPF 30 or higher daily and reapply every two hours when outdoors. Sunscreen helps prevent dark spots from worsening and promotes overall skin health.

Consult with a dermatologist or licensed skincare professional to determine the best treatment plan for your specific type of hyperpigmentation. Combination therapies, such as topical treatments combined with in-office procedures, may be recommended for optimal results.

It's important to note that treating hyperpigmentation takes time and consistency, and results may vary depending on the severity of the condition and individual skin type. Be patient and diligent with your skincare routine, and consult with a healthcare professional for personalized recommendations.

3. Aging

Cause: Reduced collagen and elastin production, sun damage, and genetic factors contribute to aging skin.

For aging skin, it's important to focus on treatments that address common concerns such as fine lines, wrinkles, loss of firmness, and uneven skin tone. Here are some effective treatments for aging skin:

Retinoids:
Retinoids, such as retinol, tretinoin, and adapalene, are derivatives of vitamin A that help stimulate collagen production, reduce the appearance of fine lines and wrinkles, and improve skin texture. Incorporate a retinoid into your nighttime skincare routine, starting with a lower concentration and gradually increasing as tolerated.

Antioxidants:

Antioxidants, such as vitamin C, vitamin E, and niacinamide, help neutralize free radicals, protect the skin from environmental damage, and promote collagen synthesis. Use a serum or moisturizer containing antioxidants daily to help combat signs of aging and improve overall skin health.

Peptides:

Peptides are short chains of amino acids that help stimulate collagen production, improve skin elasticity, and reduce the appearance of wrinkles. Look for skincare products containing peptides to help firm and plump the skin.

Hyaluronic acid:

Hyaluronic acid is a humectant that attracts and retains moisture in the skin, helping to hydrate and plump fine lines and wrinkles. Use a hyaluronic acid serum or moisturizer daily to maintain skin hydration and improve elasticity.

Alpha Hydroxy Acids (AHAs):

AHAs, such as glycolic acid and lactic acid, help exfoliate dead skin cells, improve skin texture, and reduce the appearance of fine lines and wrinkles. Incorporate an AHA exfoliant into your skincare routine 2-3 times per week to promote cell turnover and reveal smoother, more radiant skin.

Sunscreen:

Protect your skin from sun damage by applying a broad-spectrum sunscreen with SPF 30 or higher every morning, even on cloudy days. Sunscreen helps prevent premature aging, including wrinkles, fine lines, and age spots, caused by UV radiation.

Moisturizers:

Use a moisturizer formulated for aging skin to help hydrate and nourish the skin, improve elasticity, and reduce the appearance of fine lines and wrinkles. Look for ingredients like ceramides, peptides, and hyaluronic acid to help support the skin barrier and retain moisture.

Professional treatments:

Consider professional treatments performed by a dermatologist or esthetician, such as chemical peels, microdermabrasion, microneedling, laser therapy, or injectable fillers, to address specific concerns and improve skin texture, tone, and firmness.

Healthy Lifestyle Habits:

Maintain a healthy lifestyle by eating a balanced diet, staying hydrated, getting enough sleep, exercising regularly, and managing stress. These lifestyle factors can influence your skin health and contribute to a more youthful complexion.

The Importance Of Sunscreen

Sunscreen is a crucial component of a skincare routine and plays a vital role in protecting the skin from the harmful effects of ultraviolet (UV) radiation. Here are key reasons highlighting the importance of sunscreen:

Prevention of sun damage:

Uv protection: Sunscreen provides a barrier against both UVA and UVB rays. UVA rays can prematurely age the skin, while UVB rays can cause sunburn. Both types of radiation contribute to skin damage and increase the risk of skin cancer.

Reduction of skin cancer risk:

Skin cancer prevention: Prolonged exposure to UV radiation is a major risk factor for skin cancer, including melanoma, basal cell carcinoma, and squamous cell carcinoma. Regular sunscreen use helps minimize this risk.

Prevention of premature aging:

Collagen protection: UV radiation accelerates the breakdown of collagen, leading to premature aging, wrinkles, and fine lines. Sunscreen helps preserve the skin's elasticity and youthful appearance.

Prevention of hyperpigmentation:

Sunscreen helps prevent the development of dark spots, melasma, and other forms of hyperpigmentation caused by UV-induced skin damage.

Protection against sunburn:

Immediate protection: Sunscreen offers immediate protection against sunburn, reducing the risk of painful redness, inflammation, and discomfort associated with excessive sun exposure.

Maintaining an even skin tone:
Preventing uneven pigmentation: Regular use of sunscreen helps maintain an even skin tone by preventing the formation of sunspots and uneven pigmentation.

Preservation of skin health:
Barrier function: Sunscreen supports the skin's natural barrier function, preventing damage to the epidermis and maintaining overall skin health.

How to choose the right sunscreen:

Selecting the right sunscreen involves considering various factors, including your skin type, activity level, and specific needs. Choose a sunscreen labeled as "broad-spectrum," indicating protection against both UVA and UVB rays. Select a sunscreen with a Sun Protection Factor (SPF) of at least 30. SPF 30 filters out about 97% of UVB rays, while higher SPF values provide incremental increases in protection.

Opt for water-resistant sunscreens, especially if swimming or engaging in activities that cause sweating. Water-resistant sunscreens maintain their effectiveness for a certain duration even when in contact with water. Consider your skin type when choosing a sunscreen. If you have oily or acne-prone skin, choose oil-free or gel-based formulations. For dry skin, opt for moisturizing sunscreens.

Check for key ingredients such as zinc oxide, titanium dioxide, avobenzone, or octocrylene. Individuals with sensitive skin may prefer mineral sunscreens with zinc oxide or titanium dioxide.

If you're prone to breakouts, choose a sunscreen labeled as "non-comedogenic" to minimize the risk of clogged pores. Sunscreens come in various forms, including lotions, creams, gels, sprays, and sticks. Choose a formulation that suits your preference for easy and consistent application.

Always check the expiration date on the sunscreen to ensure its effectiveness. Expired sunscreen may not provide adequate protection.

Consider fragrance-free sunscreens, especially if you have sensitive skin or are prone to allergies.

Follow reapplication guidelines on the product label. Generally, it's recommended to reapply every two hours or more frequently if swimming or sweating.

Remember that sunscreen is a year-round necessity, not just during sunny days. Consistent and proper application is key to reaping the full benefits of sun protection and maintaining healthy skin.

HARNESSING NATURE: THE POWER OF NATURAL INGREDIENTS IN SKINCARE

Natural Ingredients And Their Benefits

In recent years, there has been a growing trend towards natural skincare products as people become more conscious of what they put on their skin. Natural ingredients, derived from plants, fruits, herbs, and minerals, offer a plethora of benefits for the skin without the potential side effects of harsh chemicals.

Natural ingredients offer a myriad of benefits for the skin, ranging from hydration and nourishment to protection and rejuvenation. Incorporating natural skincare products into your routine can help promote healthier, more radiant skin without the use of harsh chemicals or synthetic additives. Whether you're dealing with dryness, acne, aging, or sensitivity, there's a natural ingredient out there to address your skincare concerns.

Chamomile:
Chamomile is known for its calming and soothing properties, making it ideal for sensitive or irritated skin. It contains anti-inflammatory compounds that help reduce redness, swelling, and irritation. Chamomile also has antioxidant properties that protect the skin from free radical damage and promote healing.

Calendula:
Calendula, also known as marigold, is prized for its healing and anti-inflammatory properties. It helps soothe dry, irritated skin, promote wound healing, and reduce inflammation. Calendula is excellent for sensitive skin, eczema, and minor skin irritations.

Lavender:
Lavender is renowned for its calming and aromatic properties, making it a popular ingredient in skincare products. It has anti-inflammatory, antibacterial, and antifungal properties that help soothe and heal the skin. Lavender also promotes relaxation and stress relief, making it ideal for bedtime skincare routines.

Turmeric:

Turmeric is a powerful anti-inflammatory and antioxidant agent that helps brighten and even out the skin tone. It can help reduce acne scars, hyperpigmentation, and redness, while also providing protection against environmental damage. Turmeric is beneficial for oily, acne-prone skin and can help control excess oil production.

Rosemary:

Rosemary is rich in antioxidants and has antimicrobial properties that help protect the skin from environmental damage and combat acne-causing bacteria. It also stimulates circulation, promotes cell renewal, and improves skin tone and texture.

Aloe vera:

Aloe vera is renowned for its soothing and hydrating properties. It contains antioxidants, vitamins, and minerals that help moisturize the skin, reduce inflammation, and promote healing. Aloe vera is excellent for soothing sunburns, calming irritated skin, and combating acne.

Coconut oil:

Coconut oil is rich in fatty acids and antioxidants, making it an excellent moisturizer for dry skin. It helps to strengthen the skin's natural barrier, lock in moisture, and provide a protective layer against environmental damage. Coconut oil also has antimicrobial properties, making it beneficial for acne-prone skin.

Argan oil:

Argan oil, also known as "liquid gold," is derived from the kernels of the argan tree and is renowned for its nourishing and anti-aging properties. Packed with antioxidants, vitamin E, and essential fatty acids, argan oil helps hydrate the skin, reduce the appearance of fine lines and wrinkles, and improve overall skin texture and tone. It's lightweight and absorbs quickly, making it suitable for all skin types, including oily and acne-prone skin.

Rosehip oil:

Rosehip oil is rich in vitamins, antioxidants, and essential fatty acids, making it an excellent choice for nourishing and repairing the skin. It helps fade scars, hyperpigmentation, and fine lines, while also hydrating and soothing dry, sensitive skin. Rosehip oil is lightweight and absorbs quickly, leaving the skin feeling soft and supple.

Jojoba oil:

Jojoba oil closely resembles the natural oils produced by the skin, making it an excellent choice for balancing oil production and restoring the skin's moisture barrier. It's lightweight, non-comedogenic, and easily absorbed, making it suitable for all skin types, including oily and acne-prone skin. Jojoba oil helps moisturize the skin, regulate sebum production, and soothe inflammation.

Rose oil:

Rose oil, derived from rose petals, is prized for its luxurious aroma and skincare benefits. It has anti-inflammatory and antibacterial properties that help soothe and heal the skin, making it ideal for sensitive or irritated skin. Rose oil also has hydrating and toning effects, promoting a radiant and youthful complexion.

Squalane oil:

Squalane oil is a lightweight and fast-absorbing oil that helps hydrate, soften, and protect the skin. It's derived from olives or sugarcane and closely resembles the skin's natural sebum, making it suitable for all skin types, including sensitive and acne-prone skin. Squalane oil helps lock in moisture, reduce transdermal water loss, and improve skin elasticity.

Witch hazel:

Witch hazel is a natural astringent that helps tone and tighten the skin, minimize pores, and reduce inflammation. It has anti-inflammatory and antimicrobial properties, making it effective for soothing acne-prone skin, relieving irritation, and reducing redness.

Hyaluronic acid:

Hyaluronic acid is a naturally occurring substance in the skin that helps maintain hydration and elasticity. It has the incredible ability to hold up to 1000 times its weight in water, making it an excellent humectant. Hyaluronic acid hydrates the skin, plumps up fine lines and wrinkles, and improves overall skin texture and tone.

Green tea extract:
Green tea extract is packed with antioxidants, particularly catechins, which help protect the skin from free radical damage and reduce inflammation. It also has anti-aging properties, helps to shrink pores, and soothes irritated skin. Green tea extract is beneficial for all skin types, including oily and acne-prone skin.

Homemade Face Masks, Scrubs and Other Skincare Recipes

Simple skincare products can be made at home using natural ingredients. Here are some of the recipes to keep you beautiful.

Hydrating yogurt face mask

Ingredients:
1. Plain yogurt: 2 tablespoons
2. Honey: 1 tablespoon
3. Aloe vera gel: 1 teaspoon (optional)

Instructions:
Start with a clean face by using a gentle cleanser to remove any makeup or impurities.

In a small bowl, combine the plain yogurt, honey, and aloe vera gel (if using). Stir the ingredients thoroughly until you achieve a smooth and consistent mixture. Using clean fingers or a brush, apply the mask evenly to your face, avoiding the eye area. Relax and leave the mask on for about 15-20 minutes. Rinse the mask off with lukewarm water. Gently pat your face dry with a clean towel.

Avocado and honey mask

Ingredients:
1.   Ripe Avocado: 1/2
2.   Honey: 1 tablespoon
3.   Yogurt (optional): 1 tablespoon

Instructions:
Cut the avocado in half, remove the pit, and scoop out the flesh into a bowl. Use a fork to mash the avocado until it forms a smooth, lump-free paste. Add 1 tablespoon of honey to the mashed avocado. Honey is a natural humectant and helps to retain moisture on the skin. If you have dry or sensitive skin, you can add 1 tablespoon of plain yogurt to the mixture. Yogurt contains lactic acid, which can gently exfoliate and hydrate the skin. Mix the ingredients thoroughly until you achieve a consistent and creamy texture.

Cleanse your face and neck before applying the mask. Using clean fingers or a brush, apply the mask evenly to your face, avoiding the eye area.

Leave the mask on for 15-20 minutes to allow the skin to absorb the nourishing ingredients. Rinse the mask off with lukewarm water. Follow up with your regular moisturizer to lock in the hydration.

Benefits:
Avocado: Rich in healthy fats, vitamins (including vitamin E), and antioxidants, avocado nourishes and moisturizes the skin.
Honey: Acts as a natural humectant, attracting and retaining moisture. It also has antimicrobial properties.
Yogurt: Provides hydration and contains lactic acid, contributing to gentle exfoliation and a brighter complexion.
You can adjust the mask's consistency by adding more honey or yogurt if needed. For the most benefits, use fresh and ripe ingredients. You can use this hydrating mask once or twice a week, depending on your skin's needs.

Honey and oatmeal hydrating mask

Ingredients:
1.   2 tablespoons honey

2. 1/2 cup cooked oatmeal (cooled)
3. 1 teaspoon olive oil

Instructions:

In a bowl, mix the honey, cooled oatmeal, and olive oil until you achieve a smooth consistency. Apply the mask to your face, avoiding the eye area. Relax and leave the mask on for 15-20 minutes. Rinse off with lukewarm water and pat your face dry.

Benefits:

Honey is a natural humectant, helping to retain moisture. Oatmeal soothes and hydrates the skin. Olive oil provides additional hydration and nourishment.

Yogurt and banana hydrating mask

Ingredients:

1. 1 ripe banana
2. 2 tablespoons plain yogurt
3. 1 teaspoon honey

Instructions:

Mash the ripe banana in a bowl until it forms a smooth paste. Add yogurt and honey to the mashed banana and mix well. Apply the mask to your face, avoiding the eye area. Leave the mask on for 15-20 minutes. Rinse off with cool water and pat your face dry.

Benefits:

Bananas are rich in vitamins and moisture, promoting hydration. Yogurt adds a cooling effect and helps moisturize the skin. Honey provides additional hydration and has antibacterial properties.

Avocado and cucumber hydrating mask

Ingredients:

1. 1/2 ripe avocado
2. 1/4 cucumber, peeled and seeded
3. 1 tablespoon aloe vera gel

Instructions:

Mash the ripe avocado in a bowl. Blend the cucumber to create a smooth puree. Mix the mashed avocado, cucumber puree, and aloe vera gel in a bowl. Apply the mask to your face, avoiding the eye area. Relax and leave the mask on for 15-20 minutes. Rinse off with cold water and pat your face dry.

Benefits:

Avocado provides deep hydration and nourishment. Cucumber is refreshing and adds a cooling effect. Aloe vera gel soothes and moisturizes the skin.

Honey and aloe vera hydrating mask

Ingredients:

1. 2 tablespoons aloe vera gel (fresh or store-bought)
2. 1 tablespoon honey

Instructions:

Mix the aloe vera gel and honey in a bowl until well combined. Apply the mixture to your clean face, avoiding the eye area. Leave the mask on for 15-20 minutes. Rinse off with lukewarm water and pat your face dry.

Benefits:

Aloe vera has soothing and moisturizing properties. Honey is a natural humectant, helping to retain moisture and soften the skin.

Avocado and yogurt hydrating mask

Ingredients:

1. 1/2 ripe avocado
2. 2 tablespoons plain yogurt

Instructions:

Mash the ripe avocado in a bowl until smooth. Mix in the yogurt until you achieve a creamy consistency. Apply the mask to your face and neck, avoiding the eye area. Leave it on for 15-20 minutes. Rinse off with cool water and pat your skin dry.

Benefits:
Avocado is rich in healthy fats and vitamins, providing deep hydration. Yogurt helps moisturize the skin and has a soothing effect.

Cucumber and rosewater hydrating mask

Ingredients:
1. 1/2 cucumber, peeled and blended
2. 1 tablespoon rosewater

Instructions:
Blend the cucumber to create a smooth puree. Mix in the rosewater. Apply the mixture to your face and leave it on for 15-20 minutes. Rinse off with cold water and pat your face dry.

Benefits:
Cucumber has a cooling effect and helps hydrate the skin. Rosewater provides additional hydration and has soothing properties.

Banana and coconut milk hydrating mask

Ingredients:
1. 1 ripe banana
2. 2 tablespoons coconut milk

Instructions:
Mash the ripe banana in a bowl. Mix in the coconut milk until you achieve a smooth paste. Apply the mask to your face and leave it on for 15-20 minutes. Rinse off with lukewarm water and pat your skin dry.

Benefits:
Bananas are rich in vitamins and moisture, promoting hydration. Coconut milk is nourishing and helps soften the skin.

Avocado and olive oil hydrating mask

Ingredients:
1. 1/2 ripe avocado
2. 1 tablespoon olive oil

Instructions:

Mash the avocado in a bowl until smooth. Mix in the olive oil until you achieve a creamy consistency. Apply the mask to your face and leave it on for 15-20 minutes. Rinse off with cool water and pat your face dry.

Benefits:

Avocado is rich in healthy fats and vitamins, providing deep hydration. Olive oil helps nourish and moisturize the skin.

Strawberry and coconut milk hydrating mask

Ingredients:

1. 3-4 ripe strawberries
2. 1 tablespoon coconut milk

Instructions:

Mash the strawberries in a bowl. Mix in the coconut milk until you achieve a paste. Apply the mask to your face and leave it on for 15-20 minutes. Rinse off with lukewarm water and pat your face dry.

Benefits:

Strawberries contain antioxidants and provide hydration. Coconut milk is moisturizing and leaves the skin soft.

Egg and avocado nourishing mask

Ingredients:

1. 1/2 ripe avocado
2. 1 egg yolk
3. 1 tablespoon olive oil

Instructions:

Mash the avocado in a bowl until creamy. Add the egg yolk and olive oil to the mashed avocado. Mix well. Apply the mixture to your face and leave it on for 15-20 minutes. Rinse off with cool water and pat your face dry.

Benefits:

Avocado is rich in healthy fats and vitamins, providing deep nourishment. Egg yolk contains proteins that can help moisturize and firm the skin. Olive oil adds an extra layer of nourishment and hydration.

Papaya and yogurt nourishing mask

Ingredients:
1. 1/2 cup ripe papaya, mashed
2. 2 tablespoons plain yogurt
3. 1 teaspoon honey

Instructions:
Mash the papaya in a bowl until it forms a smooth puree. Mix in yogurt and honey to the papaya puree. Blend well. Apply the mixture to your face and leave it on for 15-20 minutes. Rinse off with cool water and pat your face dry.

Benefits:
Papaya contains enzymes that exfoliate and nourish the skin. Yogurt provides a cooling effect and adds moisture. Honey contributes to hydration and has soothing properties.

Face masks for oily skin

For those with oily skin, it's essential to use face masks that help control excess oil, reduce shine, and minimize the appearance of pores without stripping the skin of its natural moisture. These homemade face masks can help balance oil levels, refine pores, and leave your skin looking clearer and more radiant. Incorporate them into your skincare routine 1-2 times a week for best results.

Clay mask with tea tree oil

Ingredients:
1. 1 tablespoon bentonite clay or kaolin clay
2. 1-2 drops tea tree essential oil
3. 1 teaspoon apple cider vinegar (optional)
4. 1-2 teaspoons water (as needed)

Instructions:
Mix bentonite or kaolin clay with tea tree essential oil and apple cider vinegar (if using) to form a paste. Add water gradually until you achieve a smooth consistency. Apply the mask to your face, focusing on oily areas,

and let it dry for 10-15 minutes. Rinse off with lukewarm water and pat your face dry.

Benefits:
Clay helps absorb excess oil and impurities, while tea tree oil has antibacterial properties that can help prevent breakouts.

Tomato and lemon mask

Ingredients:
1. 1 ripe tomato
2. 1 teaspoon lemon juice

Instructions:
Blend the ripe tomato into a smooth paste. Mix in lemon juice and apply the mixture to your face. Let it sit for 10-15 minutes before rinsing off with lukewarm water. Pat your face dry.

Benefits:
Tomatoes contain natural astringent properties that help tighten pores and regulate sebum production, while lemon juice helps balance oil levels and brighten the skin.

Egg white mask

Ingredients:
1. 1 egg white
2. 1 teaspoon lemon juice or honey (optional)

Instructions:
Whisk the egg white until frothy. Add lemon juice or honey (if using) and mix well. Apply the mixture to your face and let it dry for 10-15 minutes. Rinse off with lukewarm water and pat your face dry.

Benefits:
Egg whites help tighten pores and control oil production, leaving the skin feeling refreshed and mattified.

Yogurt and turmeric mask

Ingredients:

1. 1 tablespoon plain yogurt
2. 1/2 teaspoon turmeric powder
3. 1 teaspoon honey

Instructions:

Mix plain yogurt with turmeric powder and honey to form a paste. Apply the mask to clean skin and leave it on for 10-15 minutes. Rinse off with lukewarm water and pat dry.

Benefits:

Yogurt contains lactic acid, which helps exfoliate dead skin cells and control oil production. Turmeric has anti-inflammatory properties to calm acne-prone skin, while honey adds moisture and fights bacteria.

For oily skin, toners are crucial for balancing oil production, tightening pores, and preventing breakouts. Here are some toners specifically formulated for oily skin to make at home:

Green tea toner

Ingredients:

1. 1/2 cup brewed green tea, cooled
2. 1/2 cup witch hazel
3. Optional: a few drops of peppermint or eucalyptus essential oil

Instructions:

Brew green tea and allow it to cool completely. Mix equal parts of green tea and witch hazel in a clean bottle. Add a few drops of peppermint or eucalyptus essential oil for a refreshing sensation (optional). Shake well before each use. Apply the toner to a cotton pad and gently swipe it over clean skin. Allow it to dry before applying moisturizer.

Benefits:

Green tea is rich in antioxidants and has anti-inflammatory properties, making it ideal for oily, acne-prone skin. Witch hazel helps control oil

production and minimize pores, while peppermint or eucalyptus oil
provides a refreshing feel.

Apple cider vinegar toner

Ingredients:
1. 1 part raw apple cider vinegar
2. 3 parts water
3. Optional: a few drops of tea tree essential oil

Instructions:
Mix apple cider vinegar with water in a clean bottle. Add a few drops of tea
tree essential oil if desired for its antibacterial properties. Shake well before
each use. Apply the toner to a cotton pad and swipe it over clean skin,
focusing on oily areas. Allow it to dry before applying moisturizer.

Benefits:
Apple cider vinegar helps balance the skin's pH levels, control oil
production, and minimize the appearance of pores. Tea tree oil has
antimicrobial properties that can help prevent acne breakouts.

Rose water toner

Ingredients:
1. 1/2 cup rose water
2. 1/2 cup witch hazel

Instructions:
Mix equal parts of rose water and witch hazel in a clean bottle. Shake well
before each use. Apply the toner to a cotton pad and gently swipe it over
clean skin. Allow it to dry before applying moisturizer.

Benefits:
Rose water helps balance the skin's pH levels, soothes irritation, and
controls excess oil production. Witch hazel tightens pores and reduces
inflammation, making this toner suitable for oily and acne-prone skin.

Homemade masks for acne-prone skin

For acne-prone skin, it's important to use masks that help unclog pores, reduce inflammation, and prevent breakouts. Here are some effective masks specifically formulated for acne-prone skin to make at home:

Honey and cinnamon mask

Ingredients:
1. 1 tablespoon raw honey
2. 1/2 teaspoon cinnamon powder

Instructions:
Mix raw honey with cinnamon powder until well combined. Apply the mixture to clean skin and leave it on for 10-15 minutes. Rinse off with lukewarm water and pat dry.

Benefits:
Honey has antibacterial properties that help fight acne-causing bacteria, while cinnamon has anti-inflammatory properties that can reduce redness and swelling associated with acne.

Turmeric and yogurt mask

Ingredients:
1. 1 teaspoon turmeric powder
2. 1 tablespoon plain yogurt
3. 1 teaspoon raw honey (optional)

Instructions:
Mix turmeric powder with plain yogurt (and honey if desired) to form a paste. Apply the mixture to clean skin and leave it on for 10-15 minutes. Rinse off with lukewarm water and pat dry.

Benefits:
Turmeric has anti-inflammatory and antimicrobial properties that can help reduce acne and soothe irritated skin, while yogurt contains lactic acid that helps exfoliate and unclog pores.

Aloe vera and green tea mask

Ingredients:
1. 1 tablespoon aloe vera gel
2. 1 tablespoon brewed green tea, cooled

Instructions:

Mix aloe vera gel with cooled brewed green tea until well combined. Apply the mixture to clean skin and leave it on for 10-15 minutes. Rinse off with lukewarm water and pat dry.

Benefits:

Aloe vera has soothing and anti-inflammatory properties that can help calm acne-prone skin, while green tea contains antioxidants that help reduce inflammation and fight acne-causing bacteria.

Face masks for aging skin

Egg white and lemon mask

Ingredients:
1. 1 egg white
2. 1 teaspoon lemon juice

Instructions:

Separate the egg white from the yolk and whisk it until frothy. Add lemon juice to the frothy egg white and mix well. Apply the mixture to clean, dry skin and leave it on for 10-15 minutes. Rinse off with lukewarm water and pat dry.

Benefits:

Egg white contains proteins and amino acids that help tighten and firm the skin, while lemon juice brightens and evens out skin tone. This mask helps minimize the appearance of fine lines and wrinkles.

Gelatin and milk mask

Ingredients:
1. 1 tablespoon unflavored gelatin powder

2. 2 tablespoons milk (you can use any type of milk, such as cow's milk, almond milk, or coconut milk)
3. Optional: 1 teaspoon honey (for added hydration)

Instructions:

In a microwave-safe bowl, mix the unflavored gelatin powder with the milk until well combined. Heat the mixture in the microwave for about 10-15 seconds until it becomes warm. Be careful not to overheat the mixture. Stir the mixture again to ensure that the gelatin is completely dissolved in the milk. Add honey to the mixture and stir until evenly distributed. Allow the mixture to cool slightly until it reaches a comfortable temperature for your skin. Apply the mask evenly to your clean, dry face, avoiding the delicate eye area. Leave the mask on for 15-20 minutes, or until it has completely dried and feels tight on the skin. Gently peel off the mask starting from the edges or rinse it off with lukewarm water if it doesn't peel off easily. Follow up with your favorite moisturizer to hydrate the skin.

Benefits:

Gelatin helps to tighten and firm the skin, leaving it feeling smoother and more toned. Milk contains lactic acid, which gently exfoliates the skin and helps to improve its texture and tone.

Honey is a natural humectant that attracts moisture to the skin, leaving it feeling soft and hydrated.

Natural scrabs for all skin types

Creating homemade scrubs allows you to customize the ingredients to suit your skin type and preferences. Here are some simple DIY scrub recipes you can make at home.

Sugar and coconut oil scrub

Mix 1/2 cup of granulated sugar with 1/4 cup of melted coconut oil in a bowl. Optionally, add a few drops of essential oil (such as lavender or peppermint) for fragrance. Stir well until the sugar is evenly coated with the coconut oil. Apply the scrub to damp skin and massage in gentle, circular motions. Rinse off with warm water and pat dry.

Sugar acts as a natural exfoliant, while coconut oil moisturizes and nourishes the skin.

Oatmeal and honey scrub

Grind 1/2 cup of rolled oats into a fine powder using a blender or food processor. Mix the ground oats with 2 tablespoons of honey in a bowl. Optionally, add a tablespoon of yogurt for added hydration and exfoliation. Stir well until a paste-like consistency is formed. Apply the scrub to damp skin and massage gently in circular motions. Rinse off with warm water and pat dry.

Oatmeal helps to soothe and calm the skin, while honey acts as a humectant to attract moisture.

Coffee grounds and olive oil scrub

Mix 1/2 cup of used coffee grounds with 2 tablespoons of olive oil in a bowl. Optionally, add a tablespoon of brown sugar for added exfoliation. Stir well until the coffee grounds are evenly coated with the olive oil. Apply the scrub to damp skin and massage in circular motions, focusing on areas of dry or rough skin. Rinse off with warm water and pat dry.

Coffee grounds provide gentle exfoliation and help to improve circulation, while olive oil moisturizes and nourishes the skin.

Sea salt and lemon scrub

Mix 1/2 cup of sea salt with the juice of half a lemon in a bowl.

Optionally, add a tablespoon of olive oil for added hydration. Stir well until the ingredients are evenly combined. Apply the scrub to damp skin and massage gently in circular motions. Rinse off with warm water and pat dry.

Sea salt provides thorough exfoliation, while lemon juice brightens and tones the skin.

Brown sugar and almond oil scrub

Mix 1/2 cup of brown sugar with 2 tablespoons of almond oil in a bowl. Optionally, add a teaspoon of vanilla extract for fragrance. Stir well until the sugar is evenly coated with the almond oil. Apply the scrub to damp skin and massage in gentle, circular motions. Rinse off with warm water and pat dry.

Brown sugar acts as a natural exfoliant, while almond oil moisturizes and softens the skin.

These scrubs are simple to make using ingredients found in your pantry and can be used 1-2 times per week to help exfoliate, moisturize, and rejuvenate the skin. Customize the recipes by adjusting the ingredients to suit your skin type and preferences.

Lip Care

Lip care is essential for maintaining healthy, comfortable, and attractive lips. Taking care of your lips ensures that they always look and feel their best, enhancing your overall confidence and well-being. Proper lip care creates a smooth and hydrated base for makeup application, allowing lip products to glide on more evenly and last longer. Dry, chapped lips can be uncomfortable and even painful, especially when they become cracked or inflamed.

There are several effective home remedies to help hydrate and soothe your lips:

Hydration: Drink plenty of water throughout the day to keep your body hydrated, which can also help keep your lips moisturized from the inside out.

Lip balm: Apply a thick layer of lip balm or lip moisturizer containing hydrating ingredients such as beeswax, shea butter, coconut oil, or almond oil. Reapply as needed throughout the day, especially after eating or drinking.

Exfoliation: Gently exfoliate your lips to remove dead skin cells and promote cell turnover. You can make a DIY lip scrub using a mixture of sugar and honey, or simply use a soft toothbrush to gently brush your lips in circular motions.

Honey treatment: Apply a thin layer of honey to your lips and leave it on fo 10-15 minutes before rinsing off with lukewarm water. Honey has natura moisturizing and antibacterial properties that can help hydrate and hea dry, chapped lips.

Coconut oil: Apply a small amount of coconut oil to your lips and massage i in gently. Coconut oil is rich in fatty acids that help nourish and moisturize the skin, making it an excellent natural remedy for dry lips.

Aloe vera gel: Apply a thin layer of pure aloe vera gel to your lips and leave it on for 10-15 minutes before rinsing off. Aloe vera has soothing and moisturizing properties that can help relieve dryness and irritation.

Cucumber slices: Place thin slices of cucumber over your lips and leave them on for 10-15 minutes. Cucumber has hydrating and cooling propertie that can help soothe dry, irritated lips.

Avoid licking your lips: While it may provide temporary relief, licking you lips can actually make them drier in the long run. Saliva contains enzyme that can break down the delicate skin on your lips, leading to increase dryness and irritation.

Humidifier: Use a humidifier in your home, especially during the winte months or in dry climates, to add moisture to the air and prevent your lip from drying out.

Protective measures: Avoid exposure to harsh weather conditions, such a wind and cold temperatures, which can further dry out your lips. Wear scarf or use a lip balm with SPF when outdoors to protect your lips from th sun's harmful UV rays.

By incorporating these home treatments into your routine, you car effectively hydrate and soothe dry lips, leaving them feeling soft, smooth and comfortable.

Lip mask recipes to try at home

Honey and coconut oil lip mask

Mix equal parts of raw honey and coconut oil in a small bowl. Optionally, add a few drops of vitamin E oil for added hydration. Apply the mixture generously to your lips and leave it on for 15-20 minutes. Rinse off with lukewarm water and pat dry.

Honey has natural humectant properties that attract moisture to the skin, while coconut oil helps to hydrate and nourish dry lips.

Shea butter and almond oil lip mask

Combine 1 teaspoon of shea butter with 1 teaspoon of almond oil in a microwave-safe bowl. Heat the mixture in the microwave for 20-30 seconds until melted. Stir well to combine the ingredients thoroughly. Allow the mixture to cool slightly before applying it to your lips. Leave the mask on for 15-20 minutes, then wipe off any excess with a tissue.

Shea butter is rich in vitamins and fatty acids that help to moisturize and soften the lips, while almond oil provides additional hydration and nourishment.

Avocado and honey lip mask

Mash half of a ripe avocado in a small bowl until smooth. Stir in 1 tablespoon of raw honey until well combined. Apply the mixture to your lips, covering them completely. Leave the mask on for 15-20 minutes, then rinse off with lukewarm water.

Avocado is rich in vitamins and antioxidants that help to nourish and hydrate dry lips, while honey provides additional moisture and promotes healing.

Cucumber and yogurt lip mask

Peel and slice half of a cucumber, then puree it in a blender until smooth. Mix 1 tablespoon of cucumber puree with 1 tablespoon of plain yogurt in a small bowl. Apply the mixture to your lips and leave it on for 15-20 minutes. Rinse off with lukewarm water and pat dry.

Cucumber has cooling and hydrating properties that help to soothe dry, chapped lips, while yogurt contains lactic acid that gently exfoliates and moisturizes the skin.

Brown sugar and olive oil lip scrub

Mix 1 teaspoon of brown sugar with 1 teaspoon of olive oil in a small bowl. Gently massage the mixture onto your lips in circular motions for 1-2 minutes. Rinse off with lukewarm water and pat dry.
 Brown sugar helps to exfoliate dead skin cells, while olive oil provides hydration and nourishment to dry lips.

These DIY lip masks can help to moisturize and nourish dry lips, leaving them feeling soft, smooth, and hydrated. Incorporate them into your skincare routine as needed to maintain healthy, supple lips.

Hands And Nail Care

Hands are often exposed to environmental stressors such as sunlight, pollution, and harsh chemicals, which can accelerate skin aging and lead to the development of fine lines, wrinkles, age spots, and uneven skin tone. Proper hand care can help minimize these signs of aging and maintain a youthful appearance.

Creating a homemade hand and nail bath is a simple and effective way to nourish and pamper your hands and nails. Here's a recipe for a soothing and hydrating hand and nail bath:

Honey hands bath

Ingredients:
1. Warm water
2. 1 tablespoon of olive oil or almond oil
3. 1 tablespoon of honey
4. Few drops of your favorite essential oil (optional, for fragrance)

Fill a small basin or bowl with warm water. Make sure the water is comfortably warm, but not too hot to avoid scalding your skin. Add 1 tablespoon of olive oil or almond oil to the warm water. These oils are rich in moisturizing and nourishing properties that help hydrate and soften the skin and nails. Add 1 tablespoon of honey to the water. Optionally, add a few drops of your favorite essential oil to the water for added fragrance and therapeutic benefits. Lavender, chamomile, or rose essential oils are great choices for relaxation and skin nourishment.

Honey has natural antibacterial and humectant properties that help to cleanse, soothe, and moisturize the skin and nails.

Soak your hands and nails in the bath for 10-15 minutes, allowing the warm water and nourishing ingredients to penetrate and soften the skin and nails. Gently massage your hands and nails while soaking to further enhance the moisturizing and relaxing effects. After soaking, pat your hands and nails dry with a soft towel.

Follow up with a rich hand cream or moisturizer to lock in hydration and keep your hands and nails soft and supple.

Sea salt bath

Ingredients

1. Warm water
2. 1/4 cup of sea salt
3. 1 tablespoon of olive oil or coconut oil
4. A few drops of your favorite essential oil (optional, for fragrance)

Instructions:

Fill a basin or bowl with warm water. Add 1/4 cup of sea salt to the warm water. Sea salt is a natural exfoliant that helps to remove dead skin cells, unclog pores, and promote skin renewal, makes your nails stronger. Stir the sea salt in the water to help it dissolve and distribute evenly.

Add 1 tablespoon of olive oil or coconut oil to the water. Optionally, add a few drops of your favorite essential oil to the water for added fragrance and therapeutic benefits. Lavender, peppermint, or eucalyptus essential oils are excellent choices for relaxation and skin rejuvenation.

Immerse your hands in the sea salt hand bath and soak them for 10-15 minutes.

This homemade hand and nail bath is a luxurious treat for your hands and nails, providing hydration, nourishment, and relaxation. Incorporate it into your self-care routine once or twice a week to keep your hands and nails healthy and beautiful.

Lemon bath

Ingredients

1. Warm water
2. Juice of 1 lemon
3. 1/4 cup of sea salt
4. 1 tablespoon of olive oil or coconut oil
5. A few drops of your favorite essential oil (optional, for fragrance)

Instructions:

Fill a basin or bowl with warm water. Squeeze the juice of one lemon into the warm water. Lemon juice contains natural alpha hydroxy acids (AHAs) that help to exfoliate dead skin cells, brighten the skin, and promote cell turnover.

Add 1/4 cup of sea salt to the warm water. Add 1 tablespoon of olive oil or coconut oil to the water. These oils are rich in moisturizing and nourishing properties that help to hydrate and soften the skin, leaving it feeling smooth and supple.

Optionally, add a few drops of your favorite essential oil to the water for added fragrance and therapeutic benefits.

Immerse your hands in the lemon and sea salt hand bath and soak them for 10-15 minutes. After soaking, rinse your hands with lukewarm water and pat them dry with a soft towel. Follow up with a rich hand cream or moisturizer to lock in hydration and keep your hands soft and smooth.

Cleopatra's Beauty Secrets

Cleopatra, the ancient Egyptian queen known for her legendary beauty, was believed to have used various natural ingredients for her skincare routine. Fortunately, some of her secrets are documented, so we can imagine what kind of cosmetics the Egyptian queen used. While the specific details are shrouded in history, there are some ingredients and practices that are often associated with her beauty regimen.

Milk Baths: It's widely believed that Cleopatra indulged in luxurious milk baths. The lactic acid in milk is said to have exfoliating properties, leaving the skin soft and supple.

Honey: Honey is known for its moisturizing and antibacterial properties. Cleopatra may have used honey as a natural humectant to keep her skin hydrated and healthy.

Oils: Ancient Egyptians, including Cleopatra, were known to use various oils like olive oil and almond oil to nourish and hydrate the skin. These oils could have been used for both cleansing and moisturizing. Fragrant oils, such as rose oil and neroli oil, might have been used for their aromatic properties. Essential oils were also used in perfumes and skincare in ancient Egypt.

Almonds: Ground almonds were likely used as a gentle exfoliant in facial scrubs. The fine particles would help remove dead skin cells and reveal smoother skin.

Natural Clays: Egyptians used various natural clays for skincare purposes. Clays like kaolin and Fuller's earth were believed to have purifying and detoxifying effects on the skin.

Herbs and Botanicals: Cleopatra might have incorporated herbs and botanicals into her beauty routine. Ancient Egyptians were familiar with plants like aloe vera, which has soothing and healing properties.

Kohl Eyeliner: Cleopatra is famous for her distinctive eye makeup. Kohl, made from a mixture of lead, copper, and other ingredients, was used to line the eyes for both cosmetic and protective purposes.

Discover the ancient beauty secrets beloved by Cleopatra herself:

Rose Water Face Tonic

This aqueous solution, infused with the essence of rose essential oil, served as Cleopatra's go-to tonic for moisturizing and revitalizing her skin. Experience the transformative effects as your complexion becomes irresistibly smooth and radiant. Simply apply rose water to your skin morning and night, or refresh throughout the day with a spritz for continuous hydration and rejuvenation.

Salt Body Scrub

 One of Cleopatra's favorite scrubs can be easily prepared at home. Take 2 tablespoons of sea salt and 3 tablespoons of heavy cream. Mix them in a deep bowl and then rub into the skin in a circular motion. Leave the scrub on the body for about 5 minutes, then wash off with warm water. The product gently exfoliates dead cells and makes the skin smooth.

Milk, Almond Oil, and Honey Bath

According to documentary evidence, Cleopatra liked to take a bath with donkey milk, almond oil and fresh honey. This was her main secret of soft radiant skin. There were even rumors that the Egyptian queen always took 3-4 donkeys with her on her travels so that she would not miss taking a bath. Of course, we will not look for donkey milk today, but this procedure can be repeated with cow's milk. Mix 100 grams of honey, 5 tablespoons of almond oil (can be replaced with olive oil) and 3 cups of milk. Pour into a warm bath. Immerse yourself for 15-20 minutes.

Hand Cream with Beeswax

Experience the velvety softness of Cleopatra's hands with this natural hand cream enriched with aloe juice and beeswax. To do this, take 2 tablespoons of aloe juice, 1 tablespoon of almond oil, 4 drops of rose essential oil, 2 tablespoons of beeswax. Melt the beeswax with the almond oil in a water bath, stir, and then add the other ingredients. When the liquid cools down, you can put it in the refrigerator. This cream is enough for a week. I hydrates and protects your hands, leaving them irresistibly smooth and supple.

Warm Hair Oils

Unlock the secret to Cleopatra's lustrous locks with this rejuvenating hair treatment. Blend olive oil and castor oil, then warm the mixture for a luxurious hair treatment. Massage the warm oils into your scalp, then indulge in 30 minutes of relaxation as the oils penetrate deeply, nourishing and revitalizing your hair from root to tip. Then wash your hair thoroughly with regular shampoo. Experience the transformative power of this ancient beauty ritual as your hair emerges silky, shiny, and irresistibly beautiful.

White Clay Face Mask

Revitalize your skin with Cleopatra's favorite beauty mask: white clay. Known for its cleansing, toning, and tightening properties, white clay is the key to achieving a radiant complexion. Simply mix white clay powder with warm water, honey, and oil to create a luxurious mask. Apply to your face, then revel in the rejuvenating effects as the mask purifies and revitalizes your skin, leaving it refreshed, toned, and luminous.

Archaeologists speculate that white clay played a pivotal role in Queen Cleopatra's legendary skincare regimen, preserving her facial complexion in immaculate condition. Rich in minerals and kaolinite, this ancient beauty remedy was believed to stimulate the production of lecithin, a vital component responsible for enhancing skin elasticity, promoting cellular regeneration, and purifying skin tissues. Versatile and effective, white clay is an ideal skincare solution for individuals with mature skin seeking rejuvenation, as well as those with dry, lackluster skin yearning for revitalization.

Blue clay has excellent anti-inflammatory and disinfecting properties, which silver owes to it. It perfectly nourishes the skin with various minerals and trace elements, tightens pores, softens and tones. Suitable for: both normal and combination skin.

Green clay - the basis of which is iron oxide. By the way, the darker the shade of clay, the more effective it is and copes with many skin problems, namely, deeply cleanses pores, normalizes the work of sebaceous glands, disinfects and dries the skin. Contraindications to this kind of "cosmetics" are pink acne. Suitable for: both oily and problematic facial skin.

Red clay - improves blood supply, removes redness of the skin, increases the elasticity of vessels and capillaries adjacent to it. The clay owes its color to the combination of red iron oxide and copper oxide. The first element gives vitality to tissues, the second promotes their elasticity. Suitable for: both sensitive and prone to irritation and redness of the face.

Yellow clay is rich in potassium and iron, thanks to which it removes toxins and saturates the skin with oxygen better than all other clay representatives. Suitable for: both flabby and wrinkled face.

Cleopatra's milk and honey face mask

Ingredients:

- o   2 tablespoons honey (preferably raw)
- o   2 tablespoons milk (you can use whole milk or any plant-based milk)
- o   1 tablespoon finely ground oats

Instructions:
In a bowl, mix honey, milk, and finely ground oats until you have a smooth paste. Apply the mixture to your face, avoiding the eye area. Gently massage your face in circular motions for a minute to exfoliate the skin. Leave the mask on for an additional 15-20 minutes. Rinse off with lukewarm water and pat your face dry.

Benefits:
Honey: Known for its natural humectant properties, honey helps retain moisture, leaving your skin soft and hydrated. It also has antibacterial properties.
Milk: Contains lactic acid, which acts as a gentle exfoliant, helping to remove dead skin cells and promote a radiant complexion. The proteins in milk can also contribute to skin nourishment.

Oats: Provide gentle exfoliation, helping to soothe and calm the skin. They can also assist in removing impurities.

Cleopatra-inspired honey and rose facial mask

Ingredients:

- o   2 tablespoons honey (preferably raw)
- o   1 tablespoon rosewater
- o   1 tablespoon finely ground almonds or almond flour

Instructions:

In a bowl, mix honey, rosewater, and finely ground almonds until you have a smooth paste. Apply the mixture to your face, avoiding the eye area. Gently massage your face in circular motions for a minute to exfoliate the skin. Leave the mask on for an additional 15-20 minutes. Rinse off with lukewarm water and pat your face dry.

Benefits:

Honey: Known for its natural humectant properties, honey helps retain moisture, leaving your skin soft and hydrated. It also has antibacterial properties.

Rosewater: Used for centuries for its soothing and anti-inflammatory properties. It can help balance the skin's pH and provide a refreshing feel.

Almonds: Finely ground almonds can act as a gentle exfoliant, promoting smooth and radiant skin. They also contain healthy fats and vitamin E, which nourish the skin.

UNDERSTANDING CELLULITE: CAUSES, TREATMENTS, AND MYTHS DEBUNKED

What Is Cellulite? Treatments And Remedies

Cellulite, often referred to as "orange peel skin" or "cottage cheese thighs," is a common concern that affects many individuals, regardless of age, gender, or body type. Despite its prevalence, cellulite remains a misunderstood and often stigmatized condition. In this article, we will delve into the causes of cellulite, explore various treatments and remedies, and debunk some common myths surrounding this cosmetic concern.

Cellulite refers to the dimpled or lumpy appearance of skin, typically found on the thighs, buttocks, abdomen, and sometimes arms. It occurs when fat deposits push through the connective tissue beneath the skin, creating a bumpy texture. Cellulite affects people of all shapes and sizes, including those who are thin or physically fit.

Causes of cellulite

While the exact cause of cellulite is not fully understood, several factors are believed to contribute to its development:

Genetics: Genetic predisposition plays a significant role in determining who is more prone to developing cellulite. If your parents or grandparents had cellulite, you may be more likely to experience it yourself.

Hormones: Hormonal changes, particularly fluctuations in estrogen levels, can affect the structure and elasticity of the skin. This is why cellulite often becomes more noticeable during puberty, pregnancy, and menopause.

Lifestyle factors: Poor diet, lack of exercise, smoking, excessive alcohol consumption, and high stress levels can all contribute to the formation of cellulite. These factors may lead to weight gain, poor circulation, and decreased collagen production, which can exacerbate the appearance of cellulite.

Aging: As we age, the skin loses its elasticity and firmness, making cellulite more visible. Additionally, the gradual loss of muscle tone and accumulation of fat deposits can further contribute to the development of cellulite.

Treatments and remedies

While there is no miracle cure for cellulite, there are several remedies and lifestyle changes that may help reduce its appearance over time. Here are some natural anti-cellulite remedies to consider:

Dry brushing: Dry brushing involves using a natural-bristle brush to gently massage the skin in circular motions. This can help exfoliate dead skin cells, stimulate blood flow, and promote lymphatic drainage, which may reduce the appearance of cellulite over time.

Coffee scrubs: Coffee grounds are often used in DIY scrubs due to their caffeine content, which can help improve blood flow and tighten the skin. Mix coffee grounds with a carrier oil like coconut oil or olive oil, and massage the mixture into the skin in circular motions before rinsing off in the shower.

Hydration: Drinking plenty of water throughout the day can help improve skin elasticity and reduce the appearance of cellulite. Aim for at least 8 glasses of water per day to stay hydrated and support overall skin health.

Healthy diet: Eating a balanced diet rich in fruits, vegetables, lean proteins, and whole grains can help maintain healthy skin and reduce the appearance of cellulite. Avoiding processed foods, excessive salt, and sugar may also help prevent fluid retention and inflammation, which can exacerbate cellulite.

Exercise: Regular exercise, especially strength training and cardiovascular workouts, can help improve muscle tone and reduce the appearance of cellulite. Focus on exercises that target the thighs, buttocks, and abdomen, such as squats, lunges, and leg lifts.

Massage: Massaging cellulite-prone areas with a handheld massager or using manual massage techniques can help improve circulation, break up fatty deposits, and reduce the appearance of cellulite over time.

Topical treatments: Some topical creams and lotions contain ingredients like caffeine, retinol, and antioxidants that claim to reduce the appearance of cellulite. While these products may provide temporary improvements, their effectiveness can vary from person to person.

Lifestyle changes: Quitting smoking, reducing alcohol consumption, and managing stress levels may also help improve skin health and reduce the appearance of cellulite.

Body wraps: Popular spa treatment that claims to reduce the appearance of cellulite by detoxifying the body, improving circulation, and firming the skin.

Myths About Cellulite

Despite being a common concern, cellulite is often surrounded by myths and misconceptions. Here are a few myths debunked:

Myth 1: Only overweight individuals have cellulite.

Reality: Cellulite can affect individuals of all body types, including those who are thin or physically fit.

Myth 2: Cellulite can be completely eliminated.

Reality: While treatments and lifestyle changes may help reduce the appearance of cellulite, it may not be possible to completely eliminate it.

Myth 3: Cellulite only affects women.

Reality: While cellulite is more common in women due to differences in fat distribution and connective tissue structure, it can also affect men.

Cellulite is a common cosmetic concern that affects many individuals worldwide. While its exact cause remains elusive, several factors such as genetics, hormones, lifestyle habits, and aging contribute to its development. While there is no definitive cure for cellulite, various treatments, remedies, and lifestyle changes may help reduce its appearance.

and improve overall skin health. By understanding the causes of cellulite, debunking common myths, and embracing healthy lifestyle habits, individuals can feel more confident and comfortable in their own skin.

Homemade Anti-Cellulite Body Treatments

Anti-cellulite body treatment you can try at home:

Coffee scrab

Ingredients:
1. Coffee grounds
2. Coconut oil or olive oil
3. Essential oils (optional)

Instructions:
Mix together 1/2 cup of coffee grounds with 2-3 tablespoons of coconut oil or olive oil in a bowl. If desired, add a few drops of essential oils such as grapefruit, lemon, or rosemary for added fragrance and potential skin benefits. Stand in the shower or bathtub to avoid a mess. Apply the coffee scrub to areas affected by cellulite, such as thighs, buttocks, and abdomen. Massage the scrub into your skin using circular motions, focusing on cellulite-prone areas. Continue massaging for 5-10 minutes to stimulate circulation and promote lymphatic drainage.

Rinse off the scrub with warm water, followed by a cool rinse to help tighten the skin. Pat your skin dry with a towel. After showering, apply a moisturizer or body oil to hydrate and nourish your skin.

For best results, use this anti-cellulite treatment 2-3 times per week.

Cellulite body wraps:

Cellulite body wrapping are treatments that claim to reduce the appearance of cellulite by wrapping the body in various materials such as herbs, seaweed, clay, or special fabrics. These wraps are typically applied to areas of the body where cellulite is most prominent, such as the thighs, buttocks, or abdomen.

The process usually involves applying a mixture of ingredients to the skin, wrapping the area with plastic or bandages, and allowing it to sit for a certain period of time, often around 30-60 minutes. Some wraps may also include additional steps such as exfoliation or massage before the wrapping process.

Clay: Clay is often used in body wraps for its detoxifying properties. It can help draw out impurities from the skin, absorb excess oil, and improve skin tone and texture.

Seaweed: Seaweed is rich in minerals, vitamins, and antioxidants that nourish the skin and promote detoxification. It is believed to help reduce fluid retention, improve circulation, and firm the skin.

Herbs: Various herbs, such as rosemary, lavender, and ginger, are used in cellulite body wraps for their soothing, toning, and anti-inflammatory properties.

Essential oils like juniper, grapefruit, and cypress are often added to body wraps for their stimulating, detoxifying, and skin-firming effects.

Clay cellulite body wraps

1. **Mix the clay powder** with water or a carrier oil until you achieve a smooth, spreadable consistency. Add a few drops of essential oils or herbs if desired.
2. **Apply to the skin:** Using a brush or your hands, apply the clay mixture to the areas affected by cellulite, such as the thighs, buttocks, or abdomen. Ensure that the skin is clean and dry before application.
3. **Wrap the area:** Once the clay is applied, wrap the treated area with plastic wrap or bandages to create compression and promote absorption. Leave the wrap on for the specified duration, typically around 30-60 minutes.
4. **Rinse off:** After the allotted time, remove the wrap and rinse the clay mixture off the skin with warm water. Pat the skin dry gently with a towel.

5. **Moisturize:** Finish by applying a moisturizer or body oil to the skin to keep it hydrated and nourished.

Seaweed cellulite body wrap

1. **Mix** the powdered seaweed with water or oil until you achieve a smooth, spreadable consistency. Add a few drops of essential oils or herbs if desired.
2. **Apply to the skin:** Using a brush or your hands, apply the seaweed mixture to the areas affected by cellulite, such as the thighs, buttocks, or abdomen. Ensure that the skin is clean and dry before application.
3. **Wrap the area:** Once the seaweed is applied, wrap the treated area with plastic wrap or bandages to create compression and promote absorption. Leave the wrap on for the specified duration, typically around 30-60 minutes.
4. **Rinse off:** After the allotted time, remove the wrap and rinse the seaweed mixture off the skin with warm water. Pat the skin dry gently with a towel.
5. **Moisturize:** Finish by applying a moisturizer or body oil to the skin to keep it hydrated and nourished.

Cellulite is a complex condition influenced by factors such as genetics, hormones, and lifestyle habits, and there is no quick-fix solution for eliminating it entirely. For those seeking more lasting results, a combination of healthy eating, regular exercise, hydration, and skincare may be more effective in managing the appearance of cellulite over time.

NOURISHING RADIANCE: THE ROLE OF NUTRITION IN ACHIEVING HEALTHY SKIN

The Impact Of Diet On Skin Health

Healthy, radiant skin is not only a reflection of external skincare routines but also of internal health and nourishment. Just as we care for our skin with topical treatments, it's equally important to nourish it from within by consuming a balanced diet rich in essential nutrients. Here we'll explore the vital role of nutrition in achieving and maintaining healthy skin, as well as the key nutrients that promote skin health.

Hydration: Water is essential for maintaining optimal skin hydration and preventing dryness and dullness. Adequate hydration helps flush out toxins from the body, plumps up the skin, and promotes a youthful complexion. Aim to drink at least 8 glasses of water per day and consume hydrating foods such as fruits and vegetables with high water content.

Antioxidants: Antioxidants, such as vitamins A, C, and E, help protect the skin from free radical damage caused by environmental stressors like UV radiation and pollution. These nutrients neutralize free radicals, reduce inflammation, and promote collagen production, resulting in firmer, more resilient skin. Incorporate antioxidant-rich foods like berries, citrus fruits, leafy greens, and nuts into your diet.

Omega-3 fatty acids: Omega-3 fatty acids are essential fats that play a crucial role in maintaining skin health and integrity. They help strengthen the skin's natural barrier, retain moisture, and reduce inflammation, which can alleviate conditions like acne, eczema, and psoriasis. Sources of omega-3 fatty acids include fatty fish (salmon, mackerel, sardines), flaxseeds, chia seeds, and walnuts.

Vitamin C: Vitamin C is essential for collagen synthesis, a protein that gives skin its structure and elasticity. It also has antioxidant properties that protect the skin from oxidative stress and promote wound healing. Incorporate vitamin C-rich foods like citrus fruits, strawberries, kiwi, bell peppers, and broccoli into your diet for healthy, glowing skin.

Protein: Protein is essential for building and repairing skin tissues, as well as for producing collagen and elastin. Incorporate lean sources of protein such as chicken, turkey, fish, tofu, beans, and lentils into your meals to support skin health and repair.

Healthy fats: Healthy fats, such as those found in avocados, olive oil, nuts, and seeds, help maintain skin hydration, flexibility, and suppleness. They also support the absorption of fat-soluble vitamins like vitamin A and E, which are crucial for skin health. Include these healthy fats in your diet to nourish your skin from the inside out.

Zinc: Zinc is an essential mineral that plays a vital role in skin health and immune function. It helps regulate oil production, reduce inflammation, and promote wound healing, making it beneficial for acne-prone and sensitive skin. Good dietary sources of zinc include seafood, lean meats, poultry, nuts, seeds, and whole grains.

Inflammation and acne: Certain foods high in sugar, refined carbohydrates, and unhealthy fats can promote inflammation in the body, which may exacerbate conditions like acne. Conversely, a diet rich in anti-inflammatory foods such as fruits, vegetables, whole grains, and omega-3 fatty acids can help reduce inflammation and improve acne symptoms.

Collagen production and elasticity: Collagen is a protein that gives skin its structure and elasticity. Certain nutrients like vitamin C, amino acids, and zinc are essential for collagen synthesis. Consuming foods high in these nutrients, such as citrus fruits, bell peppers, seafood, and lean meats, can support collagen production and maintain skin firmness and suppleness.

Gut health and skin conditions: The health of our gut microbiome can impact various skin conditions, including acne, eczema, and psoriasis. Probiotic-rich foods like yogurt, kefir, sauerkraut, and kombucha can help maintain a healthy balance of gut bacteria, which may contribute to improved skin health and reduced inflammation.

Incorporating a nutrient-rich diet into your lifestyle is essential for achieving and maintaining healthy, radiant skin. By prioritizing hydration and consuming foods rich in antioxidants, omega-3 fatty acids, vitamins protein, healthy fats, and minerals like zinc, you can support your skin's natural functions and promote a youthful complexion from the inside out. Remember that skincare is not just about what you apply topically but also about nourishing your skin from within. Embrace a holistic approach to skincare by fueling your body with the nutrients it needs to thrive, and watch as your skin radiates with health and vitality.

Top Foods For Clear And Radiant Skin

Here some of the best foods to incorporate into your diet for clear, radiant skin:

Berries: Berries like strawberries, blueberries, raspberries, and blackberries are packed with antioxidants, particularly vitamin C, which helps protect the skin from oxidative stress and free radical damage. These colorful fruits also contain fiber and water, promoting hydration and healthy digestion, which are essential for clear skin.

Fatty Fish: Fatty fish such as salmon, mackerel, and sardines are rich in omega-3 fatty acids, which help maintain skin hydration, reduce inflammation, and support overall skin health. These healthy fats also help strengthen the skin barrier, preventing moisture loss and promoting a plump, radiant complexion.

Leafy Greens: Leafy greens like spinach, kale, and Swiss chard are excellent sources of vitamins A, C, and E, as well as antioxidants like beta-carotene and lutein. These nutrients help protect the skin from sun damage, promote collagen production, and improve skin elasticity, resulting in a clear and youthful complexion.

Avocado: Avocado is a nutrient-rich fruit packed with healthy fats, vitamins E and C, and antioxidants. These compounds help hydrate the skin, reduce inflammation, and promote skin regeneration, resulting in a smooth and radiant complexion. Avocado also contains biotin, which supports healthy hair and nails.

Nuts and seeds: Nuts and seeds like almonds, walnuts, flaxseeds, and chia seeds are rich in omega-3 fatty acids, vitamin E, and antioxidants. These nutrients help protect the skin from damage caused by UV radiation and free radicals, while also supporting collagen production and maintaining skin elasticity.

Sweet potatoes: Sweet potatoes are an excellent source of beta-carotene, a precursor to vitamin A, which is essential for healthy skin cell turnover and repair. Consuming foods rich in beta-carotene can help promote a glowing complexion and reduce the appearance of blemishes and acne.

Green tea: Green tea is loaded with antioxidants called catechins, which help protect the skin from damage caused by UV radiation and environmental pollutants. Drinking green tea regularly can help reduce inflammation, prevent acne breakouts, and promote clear, radiant skin.

Watermelon: Watermelon is a hydrating fruit that contains high levels of water, vitamins A and C, and antioxidants like lycopene. These nutrients help hydrate the skin, reduce inflammation, and protect against sun damage, resulting in a refreshed and glowing complexion.

Delicious And Easy-To-Make Recipes That Will Help Support Your Skin Health

Berry Blast Smoothie

Ingredients:

- 1 cup mixed berries (strawberries, blueberries, raspberries)
- 1 ripe banana
- 1/2 cup spinach or kale
- 1/2 cup almond milk (or any milk of choice)
- 1 tablespoon chia seeds
- 1 tablespoon honey or maple syrup (optional)

Instructions:

In a blender, combine the mixed berries, banana, spinach or kale, almond milk, chia seeds, and honey or maple syrup. Blend until smooth and creamy.

Pour into a glass and enjoy this antioxidant-rich smoothie to support healthy skin from within.

Salmon avocado salad

Ingredients:
- 2 salmon fillets
- 2 cups mixed greens (spinach, arugula, lettuce)
- 1 ripe avocado, sliced
- 1/4 cup cherry tomatoes, halved
- 1/4 cup cucumber, sliced
- 2 tablespoons extra virgin olive oil
- 1 tablespoon lemon juice
- Salt and pepper to taste

Instructions:
Season the salmon fillets with salt and pepper and grill or bake until cooked through. In a large bowl, toss together the mixed greens, avocado slices, cherry tomatoes, and cucumber. Drizzle with extra virgin olive oil and lemon juice, and season with salt and pepper. Top the salad with grilled salmon fillets and serve immediately for a delicious and skin-nourishing meal.

Quinoa stuffed bell peppers

Ingredients:
- 4 bell peppers, halved and seeds removed
- 1 cup cooked quinoa
- 1 can black beans, drained and rinsed
- 1 cup corn kernels
- 1/2 cup diced tomatoes
- 1/4 cup chopped fresh cilantro
- 1 teaspoon cumin
- 1/2 teaspoon chili powder
- Salt and pepper to taste
- Optional toppings: avocado slices, Greek yogurt, salsa

Instructions:
Preheat the oven to 375°F (190°C). In a large bowl, mix together the cooked quinoa, black beans, corn kernels, diced tomatoes, cilantro, cumin, chili powder, salt, and pepper.

Stuff each bell pepper half with the quinoa mixture and place them in a baking dish. Cover the dish with aluminum foil and bake for 25-30 minutes, or until the peppers are tender.

Serve the stuffed bell peppers with your favorite toppings, such as avocado slices, Greek yogurt, or salsa, for a nutritious and skin-loving meal.

Mango avocado salad with grilled chicken

Ingredients:
- 2 boneless, skinless chicken breasts
- 1 tablespoon olive oil
- Salt and pepper to taste
- 4 cups mixed greens (spinach, arugula, lettuce)
- 1 ripe mango, diced
- 1 ripe avocado, diced
- 1/4 cup red onion, thinly sliced
- 1/4 cup chopped fresh cilantro
- 2 tablespoons balsamic vinegar
- 1 tablespoon honey or maple syrup

Instructions:
Preheat a grill or grill pan over medium-high heat. Season the chicken breasts with olive oil, salt, and pepper.

Grill the chicken for 6-8 minutes per side, or until cooked through and no longer pink in the center. Remove from the grill and let rest for a few minutes before slicing.

In a large bowl, combine mixed greens, diced mango, diced avocado, sliced red onion, and chopped cilantro.

In a small bowl, whisk together balsamic vinegar and honey or maple syrup to make the dressing. Drizzle the dressing over the salad and toss to coat.

evenly. Divide the salad among plates and top with sliced grilled chicken. Serve the mango avocado salad with grilled chicken immediately, and enjoy!

Baked salmon with roasted vegetables

Ingredients:
- o   4 salmon fillets
- o   2 tablespoons olive oil
- o   2 cloves garlic, minced
- o   1 teaspoon lemon zest
- o   1 tablespoon lemon juice
- o   1 teaspoon dried herbs (such as thyme, rosemary, or dill)
- o   Salt and pepper to taste
- o   4 cups mixed vegetables (zucchini, bell peppers, cherry tomatoes, asparagus)

Instructions:

Preheat the oven to 400°F (200°C). Line a baking sheet with parchment paper.

In a small bowl, whisk together olive oil, minced garlic, lemon zest, lemon juice, dried herbs, salt, and pepper.

Place the salmon fillets on the prepared baking sheet and brush them with the olive oil mixture.

Arrange the mixed vegetables around the salmon on the baking sheet. Drizzle with any remaining olive oil mixture. Bake in the preheated oven for 12-15 minutes, or until the salmon is cooked through and the vegetables are tender.

Serve the baked salmon with roasted vegetables hot, garnished with fresh herbs if desired.

Grilled lemon herb chicken

Ingredients:
- o   4 boneless, skinless chicken breasts
- o   Juice of 2 lemons

    o   Zest of 1 lemon
    o   2 cloves garlic, minced
    o   2 tablespoons olive oil
    o   1 tablespoon fresh thyme, chopped
    o   1 tablespoon fresh rosemary, chopped
    o   Salt and pepper to taste

Instructions:

In a small bowl, whisk together lemon juice, lemon zest, minced garlic, olive oil, chopped thyme, chopped rosemary, salt, and pepper.

Place chicken breasts in a shallow dish and pour the marinade over them. Ensure the chicken is evenly coated. Marinate for at least 30 minutes, or overnight in the refrigerator.

Preheat grill to medium-high heat. Remove chicken from marinade and discard excess marinade.

Grill chicken for 6-7 minutes per side, or until cooked through and no longer pink in the center.

Remove from grill and let rest for a few minutes before serving. Enjoy with your favorite side dishes!

Vegetable stir-fry with tofu

Ingredients:

    o   1 block (14 oz) firm tofu, pressed and cubed
    o   2 tablespoons soy sauce
    o   1 tablespoon sesame oil
    o   1 tablespoon olive oil
    o   2 cloves garlic, minced
    o   1 tablespoon fresh ginger, minced
    o   2 cups mixed vegetables (bell peppers, broccoli, snap peas, carrots)
    o   Cooked brown rice or quinoa for serving
    o   Optional toppings: chopped green onions, sesame seeds

Instructions:

In a small bowl, combine cubed tofu with soy sauce and sesame oil. Let marinate for 10-15 minutes.

Heat olive oil in a large skillet or wok over medium-high heat. Add minced garlic and ginger, and sauté for 1-2 minutes until fragrant.

Add marinated tofu to the skillet and cook for 5-6 minutes, stirring occasionally, until tofu is golden brown on all sides.

Add mixed vegetables to the skillet and stir-fry for an additional 5-6 minutes, or until vegetables are tender-crisp.

Serve vegetable stir-fry over cooked brown rice or quinoa. Garnish with chopped green onions and sesame seeds if desired. Enjoy!

Experiment with these recipes and enjoy the benefits of nourishing your skin with every bite.

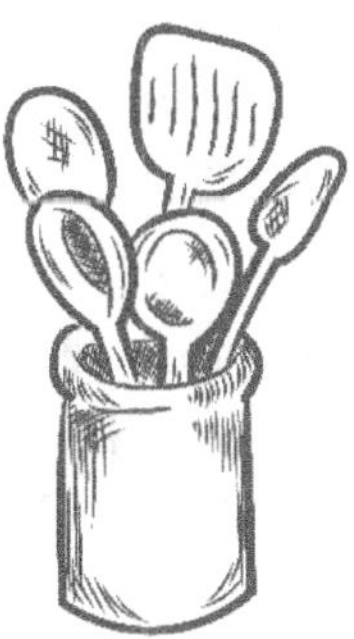

UNDERSTANDING INGREDIENTS IN SKINCARE PRODUCTS

Breakdown Of Common Skincare Ingredients

Understanding common skincare ingredients is essential for making informed choices about the products you use on your skin. These are just a few examples of common skincare ingredients and their benefits. When choosing skincare products, it's essential to consider your skin type, concerns, and sensitivities, and always patch test new products before applying them to your entire face.

Hyaluronic acid: hydrates and plumps the skin by attracting and retaining moisture, helps reduce the appearance of fine lines and wrinkles, promotes a smooth and supple complexion.

Vitamin C (ascorbic acid): powerful antioxidant that protects the skin from free radical damage, brightens and evens out skin tone, stimulates collagen production, reduces hyperpigmentation and signs of aging.

Retinol (vitamin A): stimulates collagen production, promotes cell turnover, reduces the appearance of fine lines, wrinkles, and hyperpigmentation, improves skin texture and tone, unclogs pores and prevents acne breakouts.

Niacinamide (vitamin B3): helps strengthen the skin barrier, reduces inflammation, regulates oil production, fades hyperpigmentation and dark spots, minimizes pore size, improves overall skin texture and tone.

Alpha hydroxy acids (AHAs – glycolic acid, lactic acid): xfoliates the skin by dissolving dead skin cells, promotes cell turnover, improves skin texture and tone, reduces the appearance of fine lines, wrinkles, and hyperpigmentation, unclogs pores.

Beta hydroxy acid (BHA – salicylic acid): Exfoliates inside the pores, unclogs pores and prevents acne breakouts, reduces inflammation, regulates oil production, improves overall skin texture and tone.

Peptides: Stimulates collagen production, improves skin firmness and elasticity, reduces the appearance of fine lines, wrinkles, and sagging skin, promotes a youthful and lifted complexion.

Antioxidants (Vitamin E, green tea extract, resveratrol): Protects the skin from oxidative stress and free radical damage, reduces inflammation, soothes and calms irritated skin, strengthens the skin barrier, improves overall skin health and vitality.

Ceramides: Repairs and strengthens the skin barrier, prevents moisture loss, maintains skin hydration and suppleness, reduces the appearance of fine lines and wrinkles, soothes dry and irritated skin.

Squalane: Lightweight moisturizer that hydrates the skin without cloggingpores, balances oil production, improves skin texture and tone, soothes and calms irritated skin, enhances skin elasticity and firmness.

Green tea extract: Green tea extract is rich in antioxidants, particularly catechins, which help protect the skin from free radical damage and prevent premature aging. It also has anti-inflammatory properties and helps soothe and calm irritated skin. Green tea extract is suitable for all skin types and can be found in various skincare products, including cleansers, toners, and moisturizers.

How To Read Product Labels And Choose Products Wisely

Reading product labels is essential for making informed decisions about the skincare products you use. By following these tips, you can effectively read product labels and choose skincare products that meet your needs, preferences, and skin concerns.

Understand the ingredients list: Ingredients are listed in descending order by concentration, with the highest concentration ingredients listed first. Look for active ingredients that target your specific skincare concerns, such as hyaluronic acid for hydration, retinol for anti-aging, or salicylic acid for acne treatment.

Avoid harmful ingredients: Watch out for potentially harmful ingredients such as parabens, sulfates, phthalates, and synthetic fragrances. These ingredients may cause irritation, allergic reactions, or disrupt hormone levels. Opt for products labeled as "paraben-free," "sulfate-free," or "fragrance-free" to minimize the risk of adverse reactions.

Check for allergens: If you have sensitive skin or allergies, check the product label for common allergens such as nuts, gluten, dairy, or soy. Avoid products containing these ingredients to prevent irritation or allergic reactions.

Look for multi-tasking products: Choose products that offer multiple benefits to streamline your skincare routine. For example, look for moisturizers with SPF for sun protection, serums with antioxidants for anti-aging, or cleansers with exfoliating ingredients for gentle exfoliation.

Consider your skin type: Select products formulated for your specific skin type, whether it's dry, oily, combination, or sensitive. Look for labels that indicate the product is suitable for your skin type to ensure optimal results and minimize potential side effects.

Pay attention to packaging: Consider the packaging of the product, as it can affect the stability and efficacy of the ingredients. Choose products in opaque or airtight containers to prevent oxidation and degradation of active ingredients. Pump or squeeze bottles are preferable to jars, as they minimize exposure to air and bacteria.

Check for expiration dates: Look for expiration dates or PAO (period-after-opening) symbols on product packaging to ensure freshness and efficacy. Expired products may be less effective or even harmful to the skin, so it's essential to discard them after they expire.

Read reviews and research ingredients: Before purchasing a skincare product, read reviews from other users and research the ingredients to understand their benefits and potential side effects. Look for evidence-based studies supporting the efficacy of key ingredients in addressing your skincare concerns.

ANTI-AGING SECRETS

Tips For Preventing Premature Aging

Preventing premature aging involves adopting healthy lifestyle habits and skincare practices that support skin health and vitality.

Anti-aging secrets and tips to help you maintain youthful-looking skin:

Protect your skin from the sun: Sun exposure is one of the leading causes of premature aging, including wrinkles, fine lines, age spots, and sagging skin. Protect your skin by wearing broad-spectrum sunscreen with an SPF of 30 or higher every day, even on cloudy days. Additionally, seek shade, wear protective clothing, such as wide-brimmed hats and sunglasses, and avoid prolonged sun exposure, especially during peak hours (10 a.m. to 4 p.m.).

Follow a healthy diet: Eat a balanced diet rich in fruits, vegetables, lean proteins, whole grains, and healthy fats. Include foods high in antioxidants, such as berries, leafy greens, nuts, and seeds, to help combat free radical damage and oxidative stress, which contribute to aging. Limit your intake of processed foods, sugary snacks, and excessive alcohol, as they can accelerate aging and compromise skin health.

Stay hydrated: Drink plenty of water throughout the day to keep your skin hydrated and plump. Dehydrated skin can appear dull, dry, and aged, so aim to drink at least eight glasses of water daily. You can also incorporate hydrating foods into your diet, such as watermelon, cucumber, and citrus fruits, to boost your hydration levels from within.

Get adequate sleep: Prioritize quality sleep to allow your skin to repair and regenerate overnight. Lack of sleep can lead to dull, tired-looking skin, dark circles, and fine lines. Aim for 7-9 hours of sleep per night and establish a consistent bedtime routine to promote restful sleep.

Manage stress: Chronic stress can contribute to premature aging by triggering inflammation, hormone imbalances, and oxidative damage. Practice stress-reducing techniques such as meditation, deep breathing exercises, yoga, or spending time in nature. Prioritize self-care activities and find healthy ways to cope with stress to maintain overall well-being and skin health.

Exercise regularly: Regular physical activity improves circulation, boosts oxygen and nutrient delivery to the skin, and promotes collagen production, resulting in a more youthful complexion. Aim for at least 30 minutes of moderate exercise most days of the week, whether it's brisk walking, jogging, cycling, or strength training.

Use gentle skincare products: Choose skincare products formulated with gentle, non-irritating ingredients that support skin health and resilience. Incorporate products containing retinoids, vitamin C, hyaluronic acid, peptides, and antioxidants into your skincare routine to address signs of aging, stimulate collagen production, and protect against environmental damage.

Practice good skincare habits: Follow a consistent skincare routine that includes cleansing, moisturizing, and applying sunscreen daily. Use products suitable for your skin type and concerns, and avoid harsh ingredients and over-exfoliation, which can strip the skin's natural moisture barrier and cause irritation.

Avoid smoking and limit alcohol intake: Smoking accelerates aging by depleting collagen and elastin levels, leading to wrinkles, sagging skin, and a dull complexion. Quit smoking and avoid exposure to secondhand smoke to protect your skin's health. Additionally, limit alcohol consumption, as excessive alcohol can dehydrate the skin and contribute to inflammation and premature aging.

Prioritize skincare treatments: Consider incorporating professional skincare treatments into your routine, such as facials, chemical peels, microdermabrasion, or laser therapy, to address specific aging concerns and maintain skin health. Consult with a dermatologist or licensed skincare professional to determine the most suitable treatments for your skin type and goals.

By following these anti-aging secrets and incorporating healthy habits into your lifestyle and skincare routine, you can help prevent premature aging and maintain youthful, radiant skin for years to come. Consistency, patience, and a holistic approach to skincare and overall well-being are key to achieving long-lasting results.

Recommended Anti-Aging Ingredients And Products

When choosing anti-aging skincare products, it's essential to look for ingredients that have been scientifically proven to address signs of aging and promote skin health. Below anti-aging ingredients and products to consider incorporating into your skincare routine:

Retinoids (Retinol, Retinaldehyde, Retinyl Palmitate):
Retinoids are derivatives of vitamin A that help stimulate collagen production, increase cell turnover, and improve skin texture and elasticity. They are effective at reducing the appearance of fine lines, wrinkles, and hyperpigmentation. Start with a lower concentration and gradually increase usage to minimize potential irritation.

Recommended products:
- ✓ Paula's Choice 1% Retinol Treatment
- ✓ The Ordinary Retinol 0.5% in Squalane
- ✓ RoC Retinol Correxion Deep Wrinkle Night Cream

Vitamin C (L-Ascorbic Acid):
Vitamin C is a powerful antioxidant that helps protect the skin from free radical damage, brighten the complexion, and stimulate collagen production. It can reduce the appearance of fine lines, wrinkles, and dark spots while improving overall skin tone and texture. Look for stable formulations with a concentration of 10-20%.

Recommended products:
- ✓ SkinCeuticals C E Ferulic
- ✓ Drunk Elephant C-Firma Day Serum

✓ Mad Hippie Vitamin C Serum

Hyaluronic Acid:

Hyaluronic acid is a humectant that attracts and retains moisture in the skin, keeping it hydrated, plump, and supple. It helps reduce the appearance of fine lines and wrinkles by providing intense hydration and improving skin elasticity. Look for products with various molecular weights for optimal penetration and efficacy.

Recommended products:
✓ Neutrogena Hydro Boost Water Gel
✓ The Ordinary Hyaluronic Acid 2% + B5
✓ La Roche-Posay Hyalu B5 Hyaluronic Acid Serum

Peptides:

Peptides are short chains of amino acids that help stimulate collagen and elastin production, improve skin firmness and elasticity, and reduce the appearance of wrinkles and fine lines. They can target specific aging concerns and support overall skin health. Look for products containing various peptides for maximum benefits.

Recommended products:
✓ Peter Thomas Roth Peptide 21 Wrinkle Resist Serum
✓ Dr. Dennis Gross Skincare Ferulic + Retinol Triple Correction Eye Serum
✓ The INKEY List Collagen Booster Firming Peptide Serum

Niacinamide (Vitamin B3):

Niacinamide is a multi-functional ingredient that helps strengthen the skin barrier, regulate oil production, and reduce inflammation. It can improve the appearance of enlarged pores, uneven skin tone, and fine lines while providing antioxidant protection. Niacinamide is suitable for all skin types and can be used in conjunction with other anti-aging ingredients.

Recommended products:
✓ CeraVe PM Facial Moisturizing Lotion
✓ Paula's Choice 10% Niacinamide Booster

✓ The Ordinary Niacinamide 10% + Zinc 1%

Alpha Hydroxy Acids (AHAs)

AHAs, such as glycolic acid and lactic acid help exfoliate the skin, promote cell turnover, and improve skin texture and tone. They can reduce the appearance of fine lines, wrinkles, and hyperpigmentation while enhancing overall radiance and luminosity. Start with a lower concentration and gradually increase usage to avoid irritation.

Recommended products:

✓ Drunk Elephant T.L.C. Framboos Glycolic Night Serum
✓ The Ordinary Lactic Acid 5% + HA
✓ Paula's Choice Skin Perfecting 8% AHA Gel

Sunscreen (Broad-Spectrum SPF 30 or Higher):

Sunscreen is the most important anti-aging product you can use to protect your skin from UV radiation and prevent premature aging. Choose a broad-spectrum sunscreen with an SPF of 30 or higher and reapply it regularly, especially when outdoors or exposed to direct sunlight. Look for lightweight, non-comedogenic formulations suitable for daily use.

Recommended products:

✓ EltaMD UV Clear Broad-Spectrum SPF 46
✓ La Roche-Posay Anthelios Melt-in Milk Sunscreen SPF 60
✓ Supergoop! Unseen Sunscreen SPF 40

When incorporating anti-aging products into your skincare routine, it's essential to patch test new products and introduce them gradually to minimize the risk of irritation or adverse reactions. Consult with a dermatologist or skincare professional to develop a personalized skincare regimen tailored to your specific needs, concerns, and skin type. Additionally, remember to practice sun protection, maintain a healthy lifestyle, and prioritize consistent skincare habits for optimal anti-aging results.

HAIRCARE SECRETS

Tips For Healthy And Shiny Hair

Healthy hair contributes to overall appearance and can significantly impact our self-confidence and self-esteem. Shiny, lustrous hair is often associated with beauty and vitality. Well-groomed, healthy hair can leave a positive impression and enhance social interactions, whether it's on a date, at a job interview, or during everyday interactions with friends and colleagues.

Achieving healthy and shiny hair requires a combination of proper hair care practices, a healthy lifestyle, and the use of suitable hair products. Here are some hair care secrets and tips to help you maintain beautiful, lustrous hair:

Regular washing and conditioning: Wash your hair regularly with a gentle shampoo to remove dirt, oil, and product buildup. Use a conditioner afterward to replenish moisture, detangle hair, and improve manageability. Choose products formulated for your hair type and concerns, whether it's dryness, damage, or frizz.

Use lukewarm water: Wash your hair with lukewarm water instead of hot water to prevent stripping natural oils from the scalp and hair shaft. Hot water can dry out the hair and scalp, leading to dryness, frizz, and breakage. Rinse with cool water at the end of your shower to seal the hair cuticle and add shine.

Protect your hair from heat damage: Minimize the use of heated styling tools such as blow dryers, flat irons, and curling irons, as excessive heat can damage the hair cuticle, leading to dryness, breakage, and dullness. When using heat styling tools, apply a heat protectant spray or serum to shield the hair from heat damage and reduce frizz.

Avoid overwashing: While it's essential to keep your scalp and hair clean, overwashing can strip away natural oils and lead to dryness and irritation. Aim to wash your hair no more than every other day or a few times a week, depending on your hair type and lifestyle. Use dry shampoo between washes to absorb excess oil and refresh the hair.

Trim regularly: Schedule regular haircuts or trims every 6-8 weeks to remove split ends, prevent breakage, and maintain healthy hair growth. Trimming the ends of your hair helps prevent split ends from traveling up the hair shaft, resulting in smoother, more manageable hair.

Deep conditioning treatments: Incorporate deep conditioning treatments into your hair care routine to nourish and hydrate the hair, repair damage, and restore shine and elasticity. Apply a deep conditioner or hair mask once a week, focusing on the mid-lengths to ends of the hair, and leave it on for the recommended time before rinsing thoroughly.

Protect your hair from environmental damage: Shield your hair from environmental stressors such as sun exposure, pollution, and harsh weather conditions. Wear a hat or scarf when spending extended periods outdoors to protect your hair from UV rays and environmental damage. Consider using products with UV filters for added protection.

Eat a balanced diet: A healthy diet rich in vitamins, minerals, and nutrients is essential for promoting hair health and growth. Incorporate foods high in protein, omega-3 fatty acids, vitamins A, C, and E, and biotin, such as salmon, nuts, seeds, fruits, and vegetables, into your diet to support healthy hair growth and shine.

Minimize chemical treatments: Limit the use of chemical treatments such as hair dyeing, bleaching, and perming, as they can damage the hair cuticle and lead to dryness, breakage, and dullness. If you must color or chemically treat your hair, opt for professional salon treatments and follow up with regular conditioning and deep conditioning treatments to maintain hair health.

Be gentle with your hair: Treat your hair gently to prevent damage and breakage. Avoid vigorous rubbing when towel-drying your hair, and instead, gently pat or squeeze out excess water. Use a wide-tooth comb or detangling brush to remove knots and tangles, starting from the ends and working your way up to the roots.

Homemade Hair Treatments And Natural Remedies

Hair treatments and natural remedies can help improve the health, strength, and appearance of your hair, leaving it nourished, shiny, and beautiful. Experiment with different ingredients and combinations to find the ones that work best for your hair type and concerns.

Here are some simple yet effective DIY hair treatments and natural remedies to try at home:

Coconut oil hair mask for hair growth

Coconut oil is rich in fatty acids and vitamins that help nourish and strengthen the hair, reduce protein loss, and promote hair growth. To make a coconut oil hair mask, warm up 2-3 tablespoons of coconut oil until it becomes liquid, then massage it into damp hair and scalp. Leave it on for 30 minutes to an hour, then rinse thoroughly with shampoo and warm water.

Conditioning avocado hair mask

Avocado is packed with vitamins, minerals, and antioxidants that help moisturize, condition, and strengthen the hair. Mash one ripe avocado and mix it with one tablespoon of olive oil or coconut oil until smooth. Apply the mixture to clean, damp hair, focusing on the ends, and leave it on for 20-30 minutes before rinsing thoroughly with lukewarm water.

Banana and honey hair mask for shiny hair

Bananas are rich in potassium, vitamins, and natural oils that help hydrate and soften the hair, while honey is a natural humectant that locks in moisture and adds shine. Mash one ripe banana and mix it with two tablespoons of honey until well combined. Apply the mixture to damp hair, leave it on for 30-45 minutes, then rinse thoroughly with warm water.

Apple cider vinegar rinse for oily hair

Apple cider vinegar helps balance the pH of the scalp, remove product buildup, and clarify the hair, leaving it shiny and refreshed. Mix one part apple cider vinegar with two parts water in a spray bottle. After shampooing and conditioning, spray the mixture onto your hair and scalp, massage it in, and leave it on for a few minutes before rinsing with lukewarm water.

Aloe vera hair treatment for hair growth

Aloe vera gel contains enzymes, vitamins, and amino acids that help moisturize, soothe, and strengthen the hair, as well as promote hair growth. Apply pure aloe vera gel directly to the scalp and hair, massage it in, and leave it on for 30 minutes to an hour before rinsing thoroughly with water.

Egg hair mask

Eggs are rich in protein, vitamins, and minerals that help strengthen the hair, add shine, and promote growth. Beat one or two eggs (depending on your hair length) and mix them with a tablespoon of olive oil or coconut oil until well blended. Apply the mixture to clean, damp hair, leave it on for 20-30 minutes, then rinse with cool water to prevent the eggs from cooking.

Rosemary tea rinse

Rosemary tea is believed to stimulate hair growth, improve circulation to the scalp, and strengthen the hair follicles. Steep a handful of fresh or dried rosemary leaves in hot water for 30 minutes to make a strong tea. After shampooing and conditioning, pour the rosemary tea over your hair and scalp as a final rinse.

Yogurt hair mask

Yogurt is rich in protein and lactic acid, which help strengthen the hair, hydrate the scalp, and improve overall hair health. Mix half a cup of plain yogurt with one tablespoon of honey until smooth. Apply the mixture to clean, damp hair, leave it on for 20-30 minutes, then rinse thoroughly with warm water.

Green tea hair rinse

Green tea is packed with antioxidants and catechins that help reduce hair shedding, stimulate hair growth, and add shine. Brew a strong cup of green tea and let it cool completely. After shampooing and conditioning, pour the green tea over your hair and scalp as a final rinse.

Herbal hair oil treatment for hair growth

Create a herbal hair oil infusion by steeping dried herbs such as lavender, rosemary, or chamomile in a carrier oil such as coconut or jojoba oil for several weeks. Strain the herbs from the oil and massage the infused oil into your scalp and hair, leave it on overnight, then shampoo and condition as usual.

Ayurvedic Recipes For Healthy Hair

Ayurveda, the ancient Indian system of medicine, offers holistic practices for maintaining healthy hair by balancing the body, mind, and spirit. Indian hair treatments often incorporate natural ingredients that have been used for centuries in Ayurvedic practices to nourish, strengthen, and beautify the hair. Here are some Ayurvedic practices specifically tailored for promoting healthy hair:

Hair oil massage (champi)

Regular scalp massages with hair oil are a common practice in Indian culture and are believed to promote hair growth, improve circulation, and nourish the scalp and hair follicles. Oils such as coconut oil, sesame oil, almond oil, and castor oil are commonly used for scalp massages. Warm the oil slightly and massage it into the scalp using circular motions, then leave it on for at least 30 minutes or overnight before washing it out with shampoo.

Henna hair treatment

Henna is a natural plant-based dye derived from the Lawsonia inermis plant, also known as the henna tree. In India, henna has been used for centuries to dye hair, condition the scalp, and promote hair growth. Henna treatments can add color, shine, and volume to the hair while also strengthening and conditioning it. Mix henna powder with water or other ingredients such as yogurt, lemon juice, or herbal teas to form a paste, apply it to the hair, leave it on for a few hours, then rinse it out thoroughly. Wear gloves and protective clothing to prevent staining of the skin and clothing during the application process.

Henna can leave a temporary orange or reddish stain on the skin and fabric, so take precautions to avoid contact with surfaces that may be difficult to clean. Avoid leaving henna on the hair for longer than recommended, as it may lead to overly dark or intense color results. Before applying henna to your entire hair, perform a patch test.

Amla hair mask

Amla, also known as Indian gooseberry, is a rich source of vitamin C and antioxidants that help nourish the scalp, stimulate hair growth, and prevent premature graying. Amla powder can be mixed with water or other ingredients such as yogurt, coconut oil, or henna to create a hair mask. Apply the mask to the hair and scalp, leave it on for 30-60 minutes, then rinse it out with water.

Shikakai hair cleansing

Shikakai, which means "fruit for hair" in Hindi, is a natural cleanser derived from the fruit of the Acacia concinna tree. It is used in India as an alternative to commercial shampoos to cleanse the hair and scalp without stripping away natural oils. Shikakai powder can be mixed with water to form a paste, which is then applied to the hair and scalp, massaged in, and rinsed out thoroughly.

Fenugreek hair mask

Fenugreek seeds, also known as methi seeds, are rich in protein, vitamins, and minerals that help strengthen the hair, prevent hair loss, and promote hair growth. Fenugreek seeds can be soaked overnight, ground into a paste, and applied to the scalp and hair as a conditioning mask. Leave the mask on for 30-60 minutes, then rinse it out with water.

Neem hair rinse

Neem, or Indian lilac, has antibacterial and antifungal properties that help treat scalp infections, dandruff, and other scalp conditions. Neem leaves or neem oil can be boiled in water to create a neem hair rinse. After shampooing, pour the neem rinse over the hair and scalp, leave it on for a few minutes, then rinse it out with water.

Curry leaf hair oil

Curry leaves are rich in antioxidants and nutrients that help nourish the hair follicles, prevent hair loss, and promote hair growth. Curry leaf-infused hair oil can be made by heating coconut oil with fresh curry leaves until the leaves become crispy. Strain the oil and massage it into the scalp and hair, leaving it on overnight before washing it out with shampoo.

Understanding Hair Loss: Causes, Treatments, And Prevention

Hair loss is a common condition that affects millions of people worldwide, impacting both men and women of all ages. While shedding a certain amount of hair each day is normal, excessive hair loss can be distressing and may indicate an underlying health issue. In this article, we will explore the causes, treatments, and prevention strategies for hair loss to help you better understand this condition and take steps to address it.

Causes of hair loss

Genetics (androgenetic alopecia): The most common cause of hair loss is hereditary factors, also known as androgenetic alopecia or male/female pattern baldness. This type of hair loss occurs due to genetic predisposition and hormonal changes, leading to gradual thinning of the hair and eventual baldness.

Hormonal changes: Hormonal fluctuations, such as those associated with pregnancy, childbirth, menopause, or thyroid disorders, can disrupt the hair growth cycle and lead to temporary or permanent hair loss. Imbalances in hormones such as estrogen, testosterone, and dihydrotestosterone (DHT) can contribute to hair thinning and shedding.

Medical conditions: Certain medical conditions and illnesses, such as alopecia areata, telogen effluvium, scalp infections (e.g., ringworm), autoimmune diseases, and nutritional deficiencies (e.g., iron deficiency anemia), can cause hair loss. Treating the underlying medical condition is essential for addressing hair loss in these cases.

Medications and treatments: Some medications and medical treatments, including chemotherapy, radiation therapy, antidepressants, blood thinners, and hormonal contraceptives, may cause temporary or permanent hair loss as a side effect. Discussing alternative treatment options with a healthcare professional may help mitigate hair loss associated with medications.

Stress and lifestyle factors: Chronic stress, poor nutrition, crash dieting, excessive hairstyling (e.g., tight hairstyles, heat styling), and harsh chemical treatments (e.g., bleaching, perming) can weaken the hair shaft, disrupt the hair growth cycle, and contribute to hair loss over time.

Treatment options for hair loss

Scalp massage: Regular scalp massages with warm oil can help improve blood circulation to the hair follicles, stimulate hair growth, and reduce stress. Use natural oils such as coconut oil, almond oil, or castor oil and massage the scalp gently for 5-10 minutes before washing your hair.

Nutritional supplements: Nutritional deficiencies can contribute to hair loss. Consider taking supplements containing vitamins such as biotin, vitamin D, vitamin E, and omega-3 fatty acids, which are essential for healthy hair growth. Consult with a healthcare professional before starting any new supplement regimen.

Platelet-rich plasma (PRP) therapy: PRP therapy involves injecting platelet-rich plasma derived from the patient's blood into the scalp to stimulate hair growth and improve hair thickness. This treatment may help reduce hair loss and promote new hair growth in individuals with certain types of hair loss.

Essential oils: Essential oils such as rosemary, peppermint, lavender, and cedarwood are known for their stimulating and hair-growth-promoting properties. Dilute a few drops of essential oil with a carrier oil such as jojoba or coconut oil and massage it into the scalp regularly.

Prevention strategies for hair loss

Maintain a healthy lifestyle: Eating a balanced diet rich in vitamins, minerals, and protein, staying hydrated, exercising regularly, and managing stress can help promote overall health and reduce the risk of hair loss.

Practice gentle hair care: Avoid harsh chemical treatments, excessive heat styling, tight hairstyles, and over-manipulation of the hair, as these practices can weaken the hair shaft and contribute to hair loss.

Address underlying health issues: Treating underlying medical conditions, hormonal imbalances, and nutritional deficiencies can help prevent hair loss and promote healthy hair growth. Consult with a healthcare professional for proper diagnosis and treatment.

Avoid smoking and excessive alcohol consumption: Smoking and excessive alcohol consumption can impair circulation, weaken the immune system, and contribute to hair loss. Quitting smoking and moderating alcohol intake can support overall health and hair growth.

THE MIND-BODY CONNECTION

The Impact Of Stress On Skin

The mind-body connection is a powerful phenomenon that illustrates the intricate relationship between our mental and physical health. Stress has been shown to exert significant effects on various bodily systems, including the skin.

Chronic stress initiates inflammatory responses within the body, triggering heightened production of pro-inflammatory cytokines and mediators. This cascade can worsen skin conditions like acne, eczema, psoriasis, and rosacea, while also compromising the skin's natural barrier function. Consequently, the skin becomes more vulnerable to environmental damage and moisture loss.

Prolonged exposure to stress can hasten the aging process by accelerating the breakdown of collagen and elastin fibers in the skin. This deterioration leads to the formation of wrinkles, fine lines, and sagging skin. Additionally, stress-induced oxidative stress and free radical damage contribute to premature aging, resulting in dullness and lackluster skin.

Stress disrupts the skin's healing mechanisms by impeding the production of growth factors and cytokines crucial for the wound healing process. Consequently, the recovery time for skin injuries is prolonged, elevating the risk of scarring and infection.

In addition, stress can heighten skin sensitivities, exacerbating irritation, redness, itching, and allergic reactions. Changes in the skin's immune response and barrier function further compromise its ability to fend off environmental aggressors and allergens.

Stress triggers the release of cortisol, a stress hormone that boosts sebum production in the skin's oil glands. This excess sebum production can clog pores, leading to the development of acne breakouts and aggravating oily skin conditions.

Lastly, chronic stress disrupts the skin's natural barrier function by diminishing the production of ceramides, fatty acids, and lipids vital for maintaining moisture balance and shielding against external threats. This disruption manifests as dryness, flakiness, and heightened susceptibility to environmental damage.

In essence, understanding the impact of stress on the skin underscores the importance of holistic well-being and the integration of stress-management techniques into daily life to foster skin health and vitality.

Relaxation Techniques And Self-Care Practices

Incorporate stress-reduction techniques into your daily routine, embracing practices like mindfulness meditation, deep breathing exercises, yoga, tai chi, progressive muscle relaxation, and guided imagery. These methods foster a profound sense of relaxation, effectively lowering stress levels and promoting inner calm.

Immerse yourself in regular physical activity as a potent antidote to stress. Whether it's a brisk walk, a rejuvenating jog, a refreshing swim, a spirited dance session, or a leisurely bike ride, engaging in exercise offers holistic benefits. Not only does it alleviate stress and enhance mood, but it also boosts circulation, facilitating the delivery of vital oxygen and nutrients to skin cells, thereby promoting their health and vitality.

Prioritize the paramount importance of sufficient sleep for both mind and body. Cultivate a consistent sleep schedule, aiming for 7-9 hours of restorative sleep each night. This crucial period supports the skin's regeneration, repair, and renewal processes, ensuring optimal skin health and radiance. By prioritizing adequate sleep, you empower your skin to rejuvenate and thrive, enhancing its resilience and glow.

Holistic Practices That Contribute To Overall Well-Being

Holistic practices encompass a wide range of approaches that address the interconnectedness of the body, mind, and spirit to promote overall well-being. These practices emphasize nurturing all aspects of the self to achieve balance, vitality, and harmony. Here are some holistic practices that contribute to overall well-being:

Mindfulness meditation:

Mindfulness meditation involves focusing your attention on the present moment without judgment, allowing thoughts and sensations to come and go. Practice mindfulness meditation for a few minutes each day to cultivate a sense of calm and awareness.

Deep breathing exercises:

Deep breathing exercises, such as diaphragmatic breathing or belly breathing, can help activate the body's relaxation response and reduce stress levels. Take slow, deep breaths in through your nose, allowing your abdomen to expand, and exhale slowly through your mouth.

Progressive muscle relaxation (PMR):

Progressive muscle relaxation involves tensing and then relaxing different muscle groups in the body, systematically moving from head to toe. This technique can help release physical tension and promote relaxation.

Yoga:

Yoga combines physical postures, breathwork, and meditation to promote flexibility, strength, and relaxation. Practice yoga regularly to reduce stress, improve mindfulness, and enhance overall well-being.

Tai Chi:

Tai Chi is a gentle form of mind-body exercise that involves slow, flowing movements and deep breathing. Practicing Tai Chi can help improve balance, flexibility, and relaxation.

Spending time in nature:
Spending time in nature, such as taking a walk in the park or hiking in the mountains, can help reduce stress and promote relaxation. Connect with the natural world to restore a sense of calm and tranquility.

Creative expression:
Engage in creative activities such as painting, drawing, writing, or playing music to express yourself and unwind. Creative expression can help release stress and tap into your inner creativity.

Self-compassion practices:
Practice self-compassion by treating yourself with kindness and understanding, especially during times of stress or difficulty. Practice self-care activities that nurture your mind, body, and spirit.

Digital detox:
Take regular breaks from screens and digital devices to reduce sensory overload and promote relaxation. Disconnecting from technology can help quiet the mind and restore a sense of balance.

Spiritual practices:
Engaging in spiritual practices such as prayer, meditation, contemplation, or attending religious services can provide a sense of connection to something greater than oneself and promote inner peace, meaning, and purpose in life.

Social connection:
Connect with friends, family members, or support groups to share experiences, offer support, and foster a sense of belonging. Social connections are essential for emotional well-being and stress management.

Setting boundaries:
Learn to set boundaries and prioritize your needs by saying no to activities or commitments that drain your energy or cause stress. Setting boundaries is an important aspect of self-care and maintaining balance in your life.

By embracing holistic approaches to beauty that prioritize wellness, balance, and self-care, individuals can cultivate a radiant, vibrant, and authentic beauty that emanates from within. Remember that true beauty encompasses not only physical appearance but also inner peace, confidence, and a sense of harmony with oneself and the world around us.

COMMON BEAUTY MYTHS DEBUNKED

Dispelling Common Misconceptions About Skincare And Beauty

1. *Myth: Expensive skincare products are always better.*

Reality: The price tag of a skincare product does not always reflect its effectiveness. Many affordable skincare options contain high-quality ingredients that deliver excellent results. The key is to look for products that suit your skin type and address your specific concerns, regardless of price.

2. *Myth: Cutting your hair makes it grow faster.*

Reality: Hair growth occurs at the scalp, not at the ends. While regular trims can help prevent split ends and breakage, they do not affect the rate of hair growth. Hair growth is primarily determined by genetics, diet, and overall health.

3. *Myth: You should wash your face frequently to prevent acne.*

Reality: Over-washing your face can strip away natural oils and disrupt the skin's moisture barrier, leading to irritation and potentially worsening acne. It's important to cleanse your face twice daily with a gentle cleanser suitable for your skin type and follow up with moisturizer.

4. *Myth: Tanning beds are a safe way to get a tan.*

Reality: Tanning beds emit harmful ultraviolet (UV) radiation, which increases the risk of skin cancer and premature aging. There is no safe way to tan, whether indoors or outdoors. Instead, opt for sunless tanning products or bronzing lotions for a safer, sun-kissed glow.

5. *Myth: You can shrink your pores with skincare products.*

Reality: Pore size is largely determined by genetics and cannot be permanently changed. While certain skincare products may temporarily minimize the appearance of pores by removing excess oil and debris, they cannot physically shrink or close pores.

6. *Myth: Wearing makeup every day is bad for your skin.*

Reality: Wearing makeup daily is not inherently harmful as long as you properly cleanse your skin at the end of the day to remove makeup and impurities. Choose non-comedogenic, oil-free formulas and allow your skin to breathe by going makeup-free when possible.

7. **Myth: *Plucking gray hairs causes more to grow back.***

Reality: Plucking gray hairs does not cause more to grow back in their place. However, excessive plucking can damage the hair follicle over time, leading to thinning hair or permanent hair loss. It's best to embrace your natural hair color or opt for professional coloring treatments.

8. **Myth: *Shaving makes hair grow back thicker and darker.***

Reality: Shaving does not change the color or thickness of hair. When hair grows back after shaving, the blunt ends may appear darker or coarser initially, but this is simply due to the angle at which the hair was cut. Over time, the hair will return to its natural texture and color.

9. **Myth: *You should exfoliate your skin every day.***

Reality: Over-exfoliating can damage the skin's barrier and lead to irritation, redness, and sensitivity. It's best to exfoliate 2-3 times per week using a gentle exfoliant suitable for your skin type. Listen to your skin and adjust your exfoliation frequency as needed.

10. **Myth: *Drinking more water will hydrate your skin and prevent wrinkles.***

Reality: While staying hydrated is important for overall health, drinking more water alone will not necessarily hydrate your skin or prevent wrinkles. Hydration comes from both internal and external sources, so it's essential to use moisturizers and hydrating skincare products to maintain skin hydration levels.

AFTERWORD

As we close this chapter, I invite you to carry forward the wisdom you have gained and integrate it into your daily life. Embrace the rituals that resonate with you, whether it's a simple skincare routine, a luxurious bath ritual, or a mindful meditation practice. Cultivate self-love and compassion, for it is through these acts of kindness that we truly shine.

And remember, dear reader, that the most beautiful thing about you is not how you look but who you are – your kindness, your resilience, your spirit. So go forth with confidence, knowing that you are already beautiful, just as you are.

Thank you for joining me on this journey of discovery. May your life be filled with love, light, and endless beauty.

With gratitude,

Aveline Saphino

www.ingramcontent.com/pod-product-compliance
Lightning Source LLC
Chambersburg PA
CBHW070825260726
48660CB00005B/1986